DR JOSHI'S
HOLISTIC DETOX

21 DAYS TO A HEALTHIER, SLIMMER YOU – FOR LIFE

DR JOSHI'S HOLISTIC DETOX

21 DAYS TO A HEALTHIER, SLIMMER YOU – FOR LIFE

HODDER
MOBIUS

Copyright © 2005 by Dr Nish Joshi

First published in Great Britain in 2005 by Hodder and Stoughton
A division of Hodder Headline

The right of Dr Nish Joshi to be identified as the Author of the Work
has been asserted by him in accordance with the Copyright, Designs
and Patents Act 1988

A Mobius Book

10 9 8 7 6 5 4 3 2 1

A CIP catalogue record for this title is available from the British Library

ISBN 0 340 83842 6

Set in FranklinGothic
Designed and typeset by Smith & Gilmour, London
Photography © Liberty Silver

Colour Reproduction by Dot Gradations Ltd, UK
Printed and bound by CPI Bath Press

Hodder Headline's policy is to use papers that are natural, renewable
and recyclable products and made from wood grown in sustainable
forests. The logging and manufacturing processes are expected to
conform to the environmental regulations of the country of origin

Hodder and Stoughton Ltd
A division of Hodder Headline
338 Euston Road
London NW1 3BH

The Joshi Clinic
57 Wimpole Street
London
W1G 8YP
T: 020 7487 5456
E: info@joshiclinic.com

ACKNOWLEDGEMENTS

I would like to thank my co-writer, Jane Slade, for piecing together
my thoughts, my agent, Judy Chilcote, for being a wonderful support
and friend and everyone at Hodder & Stoughton for having faith in me
not only by publishing my book but also by doing the Holistic Detox
to see that it works! Grateful thanks to Helen Coyle for her invaluable
help with pruning and for constantly guiding me away from the path of
verbal diarrhoea, my parents for pushing me and making me the person
I am, my friends for their constant support and my patients for being so
patient with me over the past year when I may have appeared distracted
or frantic. Particular thanks to Elizabeth Sanderson for all her help
and contributions, for having bottomless faith in me and for doing
the Detox again before she gets married. Also to Neil MacKichan,
Jonathan Monks, Andy Chrimes, Michelle Simms, Lilar Rashidian
and Helen Kennedy. Thank you all.

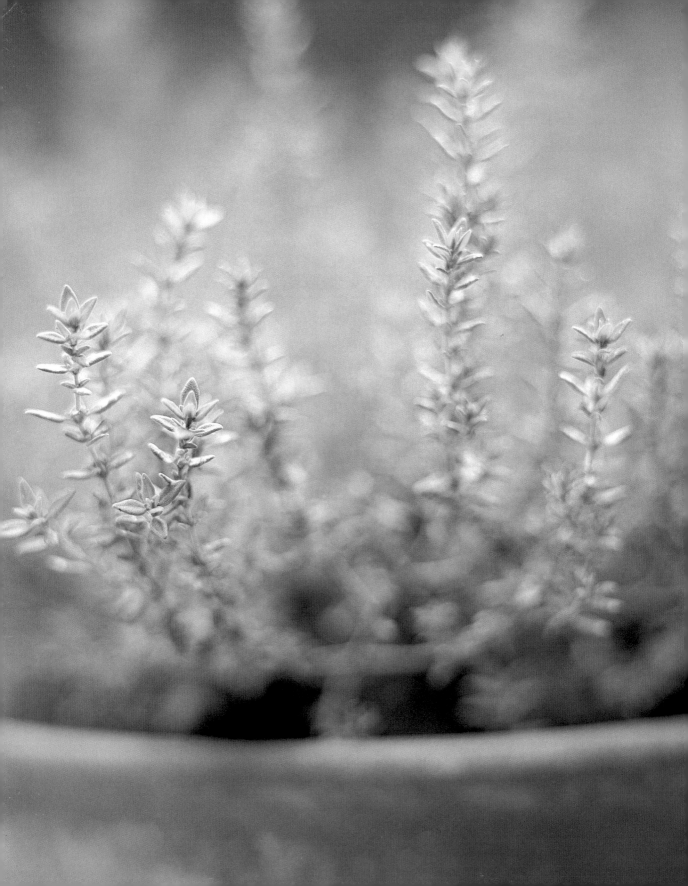

CONTENTS

INTRODUCTION

My Holistic Detox Diet, your personally tailored food plan, is rooted in the centuries-old Indian traditions of healthy eating, in the ancient science and wisdom of Ayurvedic medicine – and in both Eastern and Western approaches to 'orthodox' medicine. To this already rich mixture has been added a wide variety of healing philosophies and practices from all over the world. My search for my unique detoxing formula (and its subsequent maintenance programme) has been conducted over many years and has taken me on numerous quests and journeys.

My family is originally from Gujerat, in Northwest India, but I was born in East Africa at a time when my parents were based there on business. Then, they decided to move their business to London which is where I grew up. I was just one more small piece of hand luggage when we travelled from Tanzania to our new home in the UK.

Yet, although I was brought up in London, I was always fed a Brahmin Indian vegetarian diet. My mother had strict ideas about what we should eat and, much to my embarrassment, even campaigned for my school to provide vegetarian meals. Despite my friends constantly nipping down to the chippie or McDonalds, I never remember being tempted to join them. I actually looked forward to my mother's lentil stew, bean-curd tandoori and lemon-grass tikka. We drank plenty of water and were rarely given bread or dairy products. Generations of my family have been looked after by a family of spiritual guides – our gurus as I call them – who use Ayurvedic medicine to treat everyday ailments. So I grew up with a mother who treated my sore throats and headaches with a cocktail of herbs. I became fascinated by holistic medicine even though I grew up with a Western philospohy.

Nonetheless, the two 'D' words – 'Diet' and 'Detox' – were furthest from my mind when I completed my medical degree in Mumbai. I thought I would be an orthodox medic practising Western medicine in some capacity. It wasn't until I found myself clinical tutor at the British School of Osteopathy, with a client base made up mostly of dancers, that I grew really frustrated at the lack of response from my patients to conventional medicine. The concept of a more traditional approach, based on Ayurveda and especially on a healthy eating plan, began to loom large. These fragile creatures would hobble in to see me resembling nothing more than pipe cleaners with clothes on. It was clear that their diet of tissue paper and low-calorie drinks may have been keeping their weight down (not too many calories in tissue paper) but it provided no nutritional element whatsoever. Some of these dancers were suffering brittle bones at a terrifyingly young age and were forcing their bodies to move in ways they were neither designed nor strong enough to do.

That was when I started to crystallise the concept of Holistic Detox. I didn't want it to be about giving up foods and sacrificing the good things in life, but about getting rid of bad eating habits – like those of my dancers. Having had the good fortune to be able to spend a lot of time in my home country of India – where fresh fruit and vegetables drop from the trees, and Ayurvedic and herbal medicine are widely practised – I began to think about how these elements could be brought together in reprogramming the body to feel more energised. I also knew that ridding the body of the poisons it accumulates is not enough: mental and emotional toxins have to be flushed out too.

I asked my patients to think of their bodies as bank accounts. If you start on a lavish shopping spree – spending your body's resources heavily without putting anything back – then you find your account goes way out of balance and becomes starved of funds. If you then (like some of my dancers) start to binge on the quick-fix additives and stimulants of a very high-interest credit card, you are digging yourself into a very deep hole. This vicious splurging/bankruptcy cycle – of eating the wrong foods, craving and then bingeing – results in an emptying out of all your reserve funds and a very unhealthy body. Don't worry, however; I will show you how to get your balance back into credit.

The person who helped me consolidate my Detox Programme was Diana, the late Princess of Wales. After being introduced by a friend, Diana visited me, at the Hale Clinic and at my own private practice in London, for four years until her death in 1997. She was extremely fragile when I first met her. Her divorce from Prince Charles was going through and she felt very low and vulnerable. Diana, very anxious about the impact the divorce would have on her children, Princes William and Harry, was tired and depressed.

Initially, Diana came to see me about tension in her neck and back. It then became obvious that she needed to work on her diet if she was to find renewed energy and resolve. As an additional boost to strengthening her immune and digestive systems and purifying her blood, I gave her a remedy based on a herbal purgative devised by my mother and grandmother. Diet and remedy soon had her looking and feeling better. Diana and I quickly became friends. I frequently visited her at her apartments in Kensington Palace and she used to pop round to see me for lunch. I even taught her to make pilau rice.

The Princess was an excellent patient and conscientious about her diet. She always ate well, drank two litres of water a day, looked after herself and did plenty of exercise. After her death, I took time off to refine my Holistic Detox Programme. I was becoming ever more interested in discovering the cause of my patients' conditions rather than merely treating – and thereby masking – their symptoms. I travelled to Egypt, Eastern Europe, India and Italy to study acupuncture, herbal medicines, cupping techniques and lymphatic massage. I began to make regular visits to our family guru in Northwest India, learning from him the Ayurvedic principles of medicine that are founded on treating the whole person rather than some specific ailment. He shared with me his knowledge of herbs and how they can help as dietary supplements.

I discovered why all sorts of elements in peoples' everyday diet and lifestyle were undermining their health. For instance, I learned that fruit and vegetables bought in Western supermarkets have very little nutritional content because they are picked before they are ripe. My research also showed me that many serious illnesses are unleashed by the absorption of poisons and toxins all around us, whether these be traffic fumes, perfume sprays or pesticides, and that it is vital to be rid of them. Having formulated, on sound scientific and medical principles, the fundamentals of my Detox Programme, I then established a practice in Wimpole Street, London, with the prime aim of making it available to patients while tailoring it to their individual needs.

I have now devised a unique 21-Day Holistic Detox Programme that is healthy, safe and involves no calorie counting. This is because it is based on avoiding – as much as possible – foods that are acidic, toxic and refined, such as wheat, potatoes, red meat, alcohol and dairy produce. The idea is not only to alter the pH balance of the body from acid to alkaline (thus expelling acid toxins from the system), but also to focus on eating healthy fresh foods, restoring energy levels and losing weight.

The average Western diet is tipped far too heavily in favour of acid foods that contain chemicals which give rise to a lot of miserable conditions such as inflammation of the joints, dermatitis, muscle tensions and spasms. Balancing this acid is the first step towards ameliorating these problems and feeling much healthier. The Holistic Detox Programme achieves this by cutting down on certain foods rather than completely cutting them out. In the process, you will enter a whole new world of nutritionally healthy eating.

I have called it 'Holistic Detox' because 'holistic' means embracing the individual as a whole rather than as a collection of separate parts or (in health terms) a collage of symptoms. The Detox will, therefore, be addressing your lifestyle, diet, emotional needs, home and work environment, activity levels, external stresses – and your predisposition to certain conditions.

Commit yourself to following my Programme and I will guarantee you success on this journey. The Detox changes your palate so that you will actually dislike the taste of those foods that are bad for you – thus preventing those dreadful cravings. I guarantee you an inner and outer glow, boundless energy, a slimmer figure and, as you begin to reap these benefits, a determination not to veer from your new path of well being. If you noticed how quickly Kate Moss, Cate Blanchett and Gwyneth Paltrow, all patients of mine, regained their figures after the birth of their babies, you'll have seen how well my Holistic Detox works.

You don't, however, have to be a celebrity to benefit from this Detox Programme. Anyone who is juggling career and family, or otherwise leading a high-pressure lifestyle, can now have the body and energy levels they only previously dreamed about. My Programme is designed around the concept of thoroughly cleansing the body's 'insides' and then keeping them clean. This is a multifaceted task; after all, you wouldn't expect one cleaning product to transform your whole house. Most of us, however, offer our bodies little or nothing in the way of a clear out – and a healthy refuelling – and then we wonder why nothing works properly.

This book introduces you to a new world of foods and nutrients. It will change the way you think about food forever, both in terms of what you eat and what you cook for others. The corresponding shift in your mental and emotional approach to food will have a positive knock-on effect on your entire wellbeing.

Don't waste any more time. Make a commitment, today, to turn over a new leaf and begin an exciting journey to a fitter, slimmer, revitalised you.

CHAPTER 1
THE PRINCIPLES
OF HOLISTIC DETOX

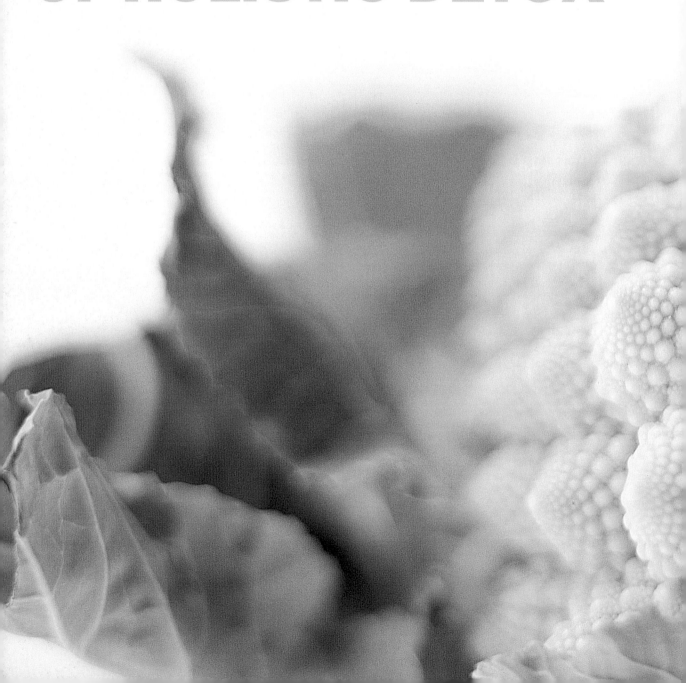

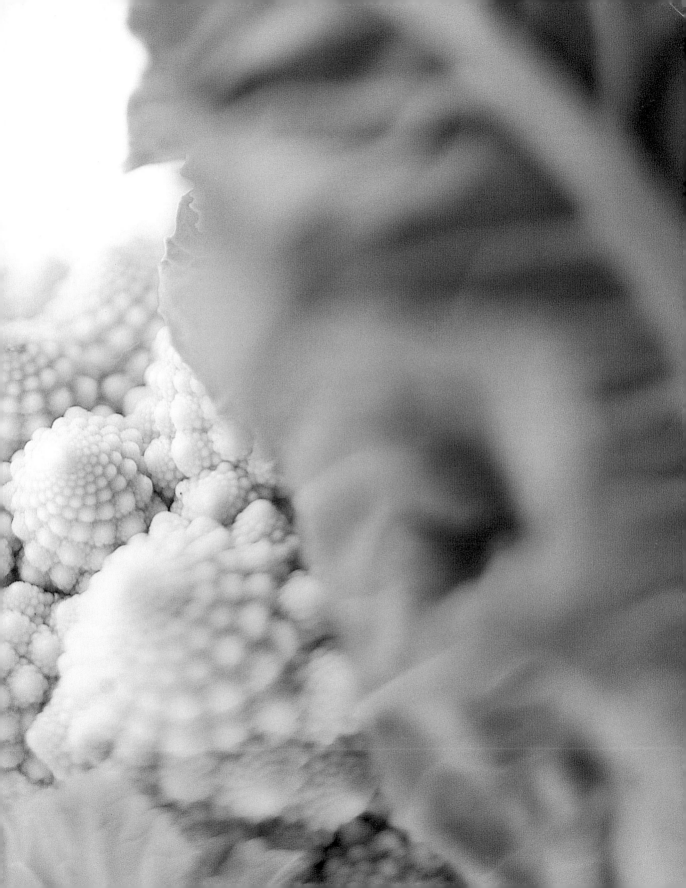

HOW OFTEN DO YOU SPEND TIME IMAGINING A NEW IMPROVED SELF – SOMEONE WHO IS SLIMMER, HEALTHIER AND FULL OF VITALITY; SOMEONE WHO LEAPS OUT OF BED IN THE MORNING FULL OF ENERGY AND COMPLETELY IN CONTROL? AND HOW OFTEN DO YOU BEGIN A NEW DIET OR EXERCISE REGIME, VOWING TO BECOME THAT PERSON, ONLY TO FALL BACK INTO BAD HABITS JUST A FEW WEEKS LATER FEELING EVEN MORE GUILTY AND DISPIRITED THAN BEFORE?

WITH THIS BOOK, YOU WILL KEEP THAT PROMISE WHICH YOU ENDLESSLY MAKE TO YOURSELF BUT NEVER QUITE FULFIL. THE JOSHI HOLISTIC DETOX PROGRAMME IS HERE TO ENSURE THAT YOU DO LOSE WEIGHT AND THAT YOU HAVE AN EVEN BRIGHTER SPARKLE IN YOUR EYE, ARE FULL OF CONFIDENCE AND LOOK AND FEEL YOUNGER AND HAPPIER THAN YOU HAVE IN YEARS.

DOES THIS SOUND LIKE A TALL ORDER IN JUST THREE WEEKS? IF YOU HAVE FOLLOWED OTHER DIETS OR DETOX PROGRAMMES IN THE PAST, YOU MAY BE SCEPTICAL – BUT I PROMISE YOU THAT THIS DETOX REALLY DOES DELIVER.

GOING ALKALINE

The Detox works because you re-establish a relationship with healthy foods. Furthermore, having learned about the toxins that beleaguer the body and the various ways of cleansing yourself to be rid of them, you will be alert to the warning signs that tell you when certain organs are not operating as they should.

By healthy foods, I mean foods that will return your body to its naturally alkaline state. My 21-Day Detox Programme is designed to alter your physical pH (acid/alkaline) balance in a way that will have a profoundly beneficial effect on the whole way your body works. Your aim is to reset your body to 'slightly alkaline' which is, in fact, your body's pH 'neutral'. Most of the time, our bodies are too acidic because of all the chocolate, alcohol, biscuits and pizza we consume – with all its sugar, salt, artificial colourants, chemicals etc.

However, neither purely alkaline nor purely acidic are desirable states so 'slightly alkaline' is where you are heading. This will enable you to eliminate the toxins in your body more easily and to break down the acidic by-products that result from the body's chemical reactions to them. These acidic deposits often lead to a sluggish digestion. Waste products then accumulate which don't all get broken down and which end up being stored as fat. Eliminating these toxins from your diet will remove a lot of stress from your digestive system enabling it to process your food more efficiently.

REPROGRAMMING YOUR PALATE

The first thing many people worry about on a detox programme is craving those foods they are no longer allowed. Remember, though, that my regime is designed to reprogramme your palate (and, consequently, your mind) to love those alkaline foods that are good for you and not to crave the acidic naughties that are so harmful.

Your first job, therefore, is to swing the pendulum in the opposite direction for a while and opt for a diet that is mostly alkaline. Not only will you then no longer crave for bread or pizza or chocolate but, in time, your digestive system will come to dislike and reject them. As order is re-established within your body, your organs will function better and your blood will flow more freely.

Don't worry; I will help you through any residual cravings during the Detox's early stages and suggests ways and foods to combat them.

Once you have taken steps to improve your internal environment, you will find that the pounds/kilos (those same ones which stubbornly refused to move in the past) start dropping off with hardly any effort and without any calorie counting. You will soon have more energy, your complexion will be clearer, nails stronger and hair glossier. In short, you will have a wonderful, radiant vitality. But you don't have to take my word for it. Your friends and colleagues will start commenting on how fantastic you look. If they don't, then you must be cheating!

CRAVINGS

A craving is the body's desire for a substance that will create a certain chemical change. Examples of such substances include alcohol, sugar, salt and chocolate. No one craves alkaline foods because, as they do not have high contents of (for instance) sugar or salt, there is nothing in them to crave. We crave acidic foods because they give the body an immediate supply of sugar/energy from an artificial source; if the body has to extricate natural glucose from fruit and vegetables, this takes a lot longer. Not all cravings are bad: a craving may be your body's cry for something it genuinely needs. Whether or not that craving becomes problematic depends on how you satisfy it.

If, for example, you regularly give your body lots of sugar and that supply suddenly stops, a chemical reaction tells the brain that your blood-sugar levels have dropped – followed by the alarm reaction: "Out of sugar! Need more sugar now!" In such cases, where you know more sugar isn't required, you need to encourage your body to be satisfied with less. You will also need to change your sugar supply to low-acid sources such as certain fruits (bananas are good) and vegetables (raw carrots are excellent).

Because we are lured into eating (nutritionally empty) acidic foods through they way they look, smell and taste, the purpose of my Holistic Detox is to change your palate dramatically so that your body is no longer interested in the extra salt, sugar, sweets and chocolates you may have been munching to excess. My aim is to reddress the balance so as to make your body more alkaline – the non-craving state.

MESSAGES FROM YOUR BODY

By listening to your body, you can learn to know what it needs. For example, two to three times a year I get a craving for orange juice. Most of the time I can't drink it because it is too acidic for me, but occasionally I will drink an entire carton without suffering any negative reaction. This is usually because my body is telling me that it is in need of vitamin C, although sometimes it is because I'm feeling a bit below par and needed something to energise me. Similarly, if I experience a mid-afternoon slump, I will get the urge to nibble on some slightly salty seeds to boost my salt levels – but will drink with them several glasses of water to keep me hydrated. If you understand how your body works, and why you eat certain foods, you can then differentiate between negative and positive cravings and are able to appreciate the effect they both have on the body. This way, you have far greater chance of maintaining a healthy disposition.

This book will show you how to use these physical signs as a basic guide to diagnosing dysfunctions within the internal organs, so that you will know whether your liver is a bit congested, your kidneys are clogged or your blood is in need of some purification. This is something alternative health practitioners have been doing for centuries. By doing it for yourself, you will begin to understand how the body works, how the digestive system behaves and how it uses the nutrients contained within different foods.

THE LIVER

Because my Holistic Detox is, in principle, a liver cleansing diet, it is helpful to understand how the liver works. Appreciating the vital role this organ plays in the digestive system will help you to look after it better.

The liver is an elaborate filtration system of cells which processes the nutrients and chemicals we absorb from our food. It has evolved over many millennia according to our diet and geographical background. People's ability to digest certain foods does, therefore, vary: it depends on what they eat, their ancestral heritage and where they live. For instance, the Japanese are better at digesting raw fish than their counterparts in the West whose systems are unused to that kind of diet. Similarly, many people from Southern Asia have difficulty in digesting meat protein because their diet is mainly vegetarian.

Certain peoples are not genetically predisposed to digesting certain kinds of food. This is why there is a growing problem with obesity in the West – because we are loading the liver with foods high in fats and chemicals that it is not used to and cannot process. Most Chinese people, on the other hand, rarely get fat even though they have a staple diet of rice. However, rice has been their main food for so long that their systems have adjusted to it – and, in any event, it does not contain the refined sugars and chemicals present in today's processed foods.

LISTENING TO YOUR LIVER

The liver, being the cleanser and filter for the blood stream, is vitally important but frequently unheeded – and abused. Our diet has changed radically over the centuries. We now eat refined foods, drink alcohol, take recreational drugs, absorb pesticides, breathe toxic fumes and spray chemicals everywhere. The liver has had to adapt to be able to deal with all these 'poisons' which is why we need to give it a break – and begin to work with it, rather than adding to its problems – if we are to prevent the onset of many chronic and debilitating illnesses.

HELPING YOUR LIVER HELP YOU

The job of the liver's filtration system is to keep the blood as pure as possible. To do this, it has to sort out the good stuff from the bad and filter off the toxins. If you nourish yourself with nutritious, freshly prepared foods, and avoid fizzy drinks, alcohol and processed foods, then you will give your liver the best chance of eliminating any poisonous chemicals that it does encounter. You'll also be giving it the time to deal with the backlog of toxins it has had to store in its own liver cells.

Another of the liver's problems is that many of the toxic chemicals that enter the body will not dissolve in water. They are fat soluble. The liver, therefore, having difficulty breaking them down, sends them to the fat stores. But until the body needs these fat cells (for conversion into energy), they will just sit there filling up with more toxins that can cause problems later. This is one of the main reasons why people find it difficult to lose weight. It is also why, during the Detox Programme, I recommend exercise – and also massage and manual lymphatic drainage – to break down the fat stores so that they are released along with the toxins.

One of the reasons I suggest avoiding fruit during my Detox is to encourage the body to convert those stored up, fatty, toxic cells into energy, rather than draw that energy from the sugar in fruit. Because it is easier to derive energy directly from sugar, the liver will always opt for that route rather than the more laborious process of converting energy from fat. This is also why many of my patients report a reduction in cellulite on my Detox, as these subcutaneous fat cells gradually get broken down.

Every drug, virus, bacterium, artificial chemical, pesticide, hormone (both taken in or self made) has to be broken down (metabolised) by the enzyme pathways inside the liver cells. This is a massive job for any organ to have to do. If your beleaguered liver becomes completely overworked and congested, it will itself eventually break down. You must, therefore, respect this vital organ and look after it. After all, you only have the one.

Cleansing the liver is fundamental to my Holistic Detox, so help this process by eating plenty of raw vegetables (40 per cent of your diet should consist of raw vegetables). Dark green leafy vegetables such as spinach, cabbage, greens and broccoli are especially good for the liver being an excellent source of the B vitamins and minerals that the liver needs to cleanse its detoxification pathways.

DETOXING SYMPTOMS

Once you start the Detox Programme, and your re-energised liver begins to release the toxins in your body into your blood stream, during the first 48 hours you may experience such symptoms as headaches, stomach pain, nausea, fatigue and even mild palpitations. If this happens, drink herbal teas with honey to maintain your blood sugar levels – and drink lots of water.

Remember too that when you have learnt how to take care of your body, your mind will also become clearer and more focused and you will feel less anxious, more relaxed and will sleep better each night. You will be ready for some wonderful ways of promoting physical and mental wellbeing – such as yoga, meditation exercises and massage.

The charts in this book, including the Cravings Box, Ayurvedic Profile Table and the BMI Index, will help you to monitor your detox symptoms and maintain your new-found vitality. As well as being fun to use, they also offer practical information about your health, personality and behaviour, give you an idea of your metabolic profile and indicate areas which may not be working as well as they should. Your goal is a healthy balance in all things, and these charts are excellent tools for learning about your own particular balance – and for keeping track of your Detox progress.

A TOXIN-FREE YOU

Your first job, on the Detox Programme, is to rid your body of all the toxins which are congesting your system, slowing down your metabolism, clogging up your digestive tract and polluting your blood. With the help of the Detox Programme, you will also be cleaning your cardiovascular system of plaque (the fatty deposits which cause narrowing and hardening of the arteries, restricting your blood flow) and working at dissolving away the calcium and mineral deposits contained within your muscles.

By combining my Diet with supplements specially chosen for their cleansing properties, you can return your body to a happy, detoxified state in just three weeks. I will also be explaining, as we go along, how these supplements work alongside amino acids, your body's own 'cleansers'. Amino acids are chemical compounds that make up the proteins needed to build all living cells. They also play a vital role in purifying your organs and helping you re-establish a normal metabolism. Vitamins are another essential element in the optimum functioning of your metabolism. To be assured of a thorough spring clean, everything must be working well together.

At the end of the 21-Day Detox, you can expect to be rid of mood swings and lethargy, you will feel revitalised, have a refreshed and replenished energy store and a new spring in your step. Because your whole internal landscape will be so much cleaner, nutrients will be able – far more quickly and efficiently – to reach and nourish your organs, muscles and brain. One of the results will be a greater clarity of thought which will enable you to take control of all the external factors in your life (work, family, friends etc.) and

cope much better with the constant demands of today's fast-paced world.

The case histories from my patients will show you how far reaching the effects of the Detox Programme can be. Read how their physical health was transformed – as was their mental attitude towards their lives, health, happiness, work stress, and relationships. Their stories will be found throughout the book and are there to help motivate you, keep you on track and, in some instances, provide useful examples of shared symptoms and tendencies.

Life is about creating positive changes and I want to show you how, in three short weeks, you can make lasting changes that will greatly improve and enhance your life's potential and create a much calmer, more peaceful and more organised you.

BEATING THE FOOD DEMONS

Three weeks is not a long time to abstain from alcohol, saturated fats, sugars, cakes and chocolates. I don't deny that you may have moments of weakness, but I will show you how to cope with those. The essential point is to make a three-week commitment to adjusting your dietary intake so as to avoid potentially addictive foods.

We are not addicted to lettuce or celery or foods that are good for us but, unfortunately, we do become addicted to foods that are toxic and potentially dangerous. The Detox sets out the way for you to retrain your body to overcome these addictions. This is not a journey of self-sacrifice and pain. We are going to work together, devoting three weeks to the job. I am not saying that you will never be able to eat pizza and cakes or drink wine ever again, but that this three-week

Programme will set you on a course that will prepare you for the next stage – the Maintenance Programme – where a greater variety of foods will be reintroduced into your diet. This Maintenance Programme will help you to deal with the effects of eating a slice of pizza, a slice of cake or drinking a glass of wine without feeling guilty and without it having a detrimental effect on your system.

The 21-Day Holistic Detox reconditions your body so that you can eat the occasional 'naughty' without causing problems. The odd pizza or cake can easily be digested and eliminated without causing stagnation or weight gain. It is not going to clutter up your colon or congeal and adhere to your digestive tract – unless you overdo it, of course.

ADDICTIONS

An addiction is very different from a craving. Whereas a craving is a temporary state, an addiction is a long term, habitual problem. We create an addiction by giving our bodies high levels of certain elements associated with such things as cigarettes, coffee, many alcoholic drinks, sweets, biscuits and cakes. Often we do not even feel we want to give our bodies these things, but they have become a habit. Having a drink or chocolate every day is a form of addiction. Addictive foods give us an immediate 'hit' of feeling relaxed, comfortable, happy, confidant and transported. Try to imagine how much you would miss that drink or bar of

chocolate if you could not have it – and that's the measure of your addiction.

We tend to be addicted to food that is artificially coloured and sweetened: it looks bright, alluring and attractive, it has a pleasant texture (we all know how lovely melted chocolate feels as well as tastes) and tastes intoxicating. It is hard to argue that alkaline foods – such as vegetables, chicken and fish – have the same qualities. Most are mild-tasting sources of natural energy, which is why we like to pep them up by adding salt and pepper and spicy sauces. However, it is important to wean yourself off your addictions so that your body becomes used to lower levels of polluting toxins and can revert to extracting the sugar/energy it needs from natural sources.

FRESH FOOD IS BEST

My Detox Programme will rid your system of the
toxins and poisons that it has accumulated over
many years. I don't just mean the internal build
up of waste matter that is ingested with food, but
also the effects of environmental pollution on the
body. To this end, you need to be thinking about
the nutrient value of the food you are actually
putting in your mouth. Too many of us rely on
supermarket convenience foods that have little
nutritional value and are packaged in plastics
that are themselves full of toxins and chemicals.

Intensive farming, nowadays a widespread
practice, also poses food problems. It often
involves the use of artificial and chemical
stimulants, and/or genetic engineering, and
while this may result in vast quantities of food
being produced more quickly, there is a greater
likelihood of that food being devoid of nutritional
value and producing a build up of toxins in the
body. Furthermore, the fruit, vegetables, chicken
etc. that you see on the shelves may have crossed
continents and oceans before reaching the store.
They are, therefore, not fresh and their nutrient
levels are that much lower.

I try to encourage my patients to eat, as
far as possible, freshly prepared meals from
food that is either in season and grown locally
(which means the vitamin and mineral content
will be considerably higher) or food that is grown
as organically as possible. However, don't be
mistaken by thinking that 'organic' necessarily
means 'pure and toxin-free'. The situation
is more complex than that.

ORGANIC AND BIODYNAMIC

Although vegetables may be grown organically
in the UK, this does not mean that the farmer has
total control over the quality of his animal manure
or organic fertiliser. For example, the water
consumed by cows in the streams and rivers may
be full of heavy metals and other toxins produced
by chemical factories. Toxic animal manure may
then be used as an organic fertiliser for organic
foods. In the UK, The Soil Association monitors
organic food using very strict guidelines but the
same is not always true for organic associations
in other countries. This is why it is essential to
wash everything, even organic produce, before
eating it.

Biodynamic produce, which is increasing
in popularity, is better (see Chapter 2) because
it is grown and fed using a holistic system: all
the meats, fruits and vegetables produced
are a product of the farm itself with no outside
additives, manures or pesticides. There are
several farms, spread around the country,
that have retail outlets on site, and some
supermarkets stock produce grown by
biodynamic methods.

WATER = VITALITY

Water is another area that is commonly misunderstood. Most of us believe that the quantity of water drunk is what's important – and I do recommend that you consume at least two litres a day. But you must also be aware of the quality of that water. I advise my patients to buy a water filter. Mineral water has been left in plastic bottles for too long (it can sometimes be stored in warehouses for up to two years) so the chemicals (such as PCBs which can cause hormonal disorders) from the packaging may leach into it. Tap water (which has been recycled and filtered many times) has not been tested for certain chemicals that could be very toxic, for example hormones from the contraceptive pill.

Water is also an important element of the fish we eat. Companies, as a by-product of their manufacturing process, are dumping many chemicals into rivers, streams or the sea and these will produce high levels of toxic waste. While farmed organic fish is extremely good for us, we should only eat smaller amounts of the larger marine fish, such as tuna, because of their very high levels of the 'heavy metals' mercury and lead. Avoid, too, shellfish such as oysters and mussels: their nickname – the 'scavengers of the seabed' – explains why!

It can be incredibly difficult for the body to expel heavy metals, particularly if it has ingested high levels of lead or mercury, for example, over a period of time. Because they have no natural metabolic pathway (the chemical channel that allows them to be broken down and eliminated), these substances end up being stored in the body's fat cells or organs, where they disrupt organ function which may contribute to infertility or memory loss.

LIVING IN A POLLUTED WORLD

We all know about car fumes and air pollution, but many of us don't realise that perfume sprays, furniture polishes, make up, washing detergents and other everyday items contain substances that are toxic and can be responsible for making us feel lethargic and generally unwell, as well as ageing us prematurely.

That lovely pine-fresh smell and orange glow emanating from your wooden chest or floor is nothing more than harmful chemical vapours which, if they enter your system, will start to deplete your metabolic functioning and make you ill. The long-term effect of amalgam fillings in your teeth can cause heavy-metal poisoning which, while it might not be evident for many years, could eventually lead to impaired nerve function.

Scientific studies have shown that people who cook with aluminium saucepans and utensils have higher chance of developing Alzheimer's because the aluminium (not only in the food, but also as a vapour coming off a hot saucepan) enters the bloodstream and eventually makes its way into the blood supply of the brain. There, it is absorbed into the cerebrospinal fluid and causes amyloidal plaques (deposits of aluminium silicate) within the brain tissue that dramatically inhibit certain cells critical to memory and learning. These plaques can eventually lead to Alzheimer's and other conditions causing mental impairment.

Every year, we create thousands more poisons, toxins and chemicals that are dangerous to the body. Their purpose is to speed up and make more efficient the tasks of cleaning, cooking, travelling, producing food and communicating via mobile phones, but they also greatly increase the amount of chemicals that we eat, drink, breathe and otherwise ingest. Nowadays, because there are so many of them, they can quickly accumulate to a toxic level.

Every chemical process in the body – and we have tens of millions of such processes happening every minute – produces toxins as an end result, and these waste products need to be eliminated from the body and eliminated effectively. If they are not, then the toxins will be stored and the effects of them will build up over time. Primarily they will simply make our bodies tired and sluggish; but eventually, if not cleaned out, they will result in problems of all kinds – impaired kidney function, gallstones, increased hyperacidity (and, therefore, ulcers) and, finally, a deeply depressed immune system.

FIGHTING THE ENEMY

Although the toxicity of our environment sounds terribly alarming, the good news is that the human immune system (our main method of fighting off threats to the body) is incredibly robust and very good at dealing with many of these poisons. The body also has its complex excretory system whereby it can eliminate toxins – through breathing, sweating, urinating and defecating. It is only when these elimination processes are impaired or compromised that we accumulate toxins in the body and have to endure the resultant debilitating symptoms.

Problems arise when you are in contact with toxins all the time, ingesting them bit-by-bit, often in minute amounts. It is their cumulative effect over a long period of time that is dangerous and can eat away at the body's strength and core stability. If combined with stress, irregular sleeping patterns and eating hollow foods, the toxin will start to weaken your body, thus making it more prone to disease. Strong and efficient though your immune and excretory systems are, you probably have (most of us do) a body that is suffering from toxic overload and are desperately in need of this Detox.

How often, then, should you detox? If you are constantly absorbing these toxins, you need to be getting rid of them just as frequently. Should detox be a way of life? Yes, it should. If you have thoroughly cleansed your body but you are still exposing it to the same pollutants as before then, every so often, you need to embark on an internal spring-clean to remove all the particularly stubborn toxins.

A concentrated, deep-cleansing detox once or twice a year will keep your body's level of toxicity under control and ensure that the more intransigent toxins are eliminated. You'll notice the difference: as your bodily functions improve, you will, for instance, suffer far less feeling bloated or tired and those headaches will most probably vanish. Your digestive process will improve, your liver and kidneys will function more effectively, your blood will purify itself more easily and your hormone levels will find their perfect balance.

The effect of this Detox is to allow your body to cope with external evils more easily; but, to achieve that, you have to stop putting them into your body in the first place. Because you can do nothing about toxins such as traffic fumes, over which you have no control, the basis of the Detox is to eliminate most of the toxins you ingest for a minimum period of three weeks. This has the effect of giving your body a rest from struggling to digest and eliminate poisons and also helping it to remove those already stored.

DEALING WITH CHEMICALS

My Holistic Detox is a twofold process.
First: you are going to alter the habits (eating, drinking and smoking) through which we all abuse our bodies and thereby create those symptoms of sluggishness, tiredness, hormonal imbalances, aching joints, headaches etc. This means eliminating potentially harmful toxins from your diet.

Second: you are also going to ensure that you use fewer chemicals in your make-up, homes, workplace, car, etc. You know that CFCs (those chemicals containing atoms of carbon, fluoride and chlorine which are daily released by such objects as hairsprays) are doing untold damage to the ozone layer, so imagine what they must be doing to your liver!

There are plenty of simple steps to take to minimise the damage. One of the easiest ways of reducing toxins coming into the house is by taking your shoes off and leaving them at the door. Studies have shown that one of the main transporters of lead into the home is the shoe. It is extraordinary how seldom we think about the toxic-laden tarmac, dirt and other unknown substances found in the street that we pick up on the soles of our shoes and then cheerfully distribute through the home.

Preventing chemicals being absorbed

An air purifier or humidifier or ioniser helps to filter impurities from the air you breathe, but even opening a window in your bedroom at night will make a big difference. Keeping the windows shut means you will be breathing in stagnant, polluted air for eight hours. Opening them will allow the circulation of fresher, less-polluted air during the hours of reduced, night-time traffic. There are natural cleaning products that will reduce the amount of chemical fumes that you inhale, and natural detergents that will reduce the amount of chemicals being absorbed by your skin through your clothes and sheets. If the detergent is biodegradable, it also means that your body is able to process and eliminate whatever chemicals are used. This is most important for washing sheets and bedding because of the amount of time you spend sleeping in close contact with your sheets and duvet covers, as anybody who has ever developed a rash after changing their detergent will know. Avoiding a toxic bedtime environment also allows your body to recover from all the toxins it has been exposed to during the day.

These are all very easy lifestyle changes to make yet they will have an enormous effect on your wellbeing. By reducing the amount of poison that you eat, inhale and absorb every day, and by cleaning out the toxins that are already stored within your body, you will vastly improve your elimination pathways. This, in turn, will allow your body to cope better with both its internal and external environment, keeping itself healthier and thereby reducing the potential risk of disease.

DETOX SUPPLEMENTS

It is not essential to supplement your diet with herbal preparations or vitamins while on the Detox. They may, however, help you progress a little faster, and give your body the boost it needs, particularly if you are feeling lethargic, suffering from bloating and finding it hard to shift excess weight. Most of the vitamins and supplements I talk about are readily available from health-food shops, high-street chemists, nutritional websites and homeopathic outlets – as well as occurring in many foods.

For the purposes of the Detox, there are three major families of supplements of particular interest: amino acids, antioxidants and digestive aids.

AMINO ACIDS

Amino acids are essential to make all cells, hormones and enzymes, and are used by the body to repair and maintain muscle tissue and nerve fibre. Amino acids are found in such proteins as chicken, fish, eggs and soya products.

GLUTAMINE: important for muscle growth and nourishment and for preventing muscle tissue breakdown (anti-proteolytic). Helps maintain the correct acid/alkaline balance of the body. Promotes mental clarity and a healthy digestive tract. Found in protein such as fish, meat and beans.

CHOLINE AND INOSITOL: good for liver cleansing, formation of lecithin, metabolising fat, gall bladder and kidneys, also brain function, stress reduction. A report published in the *Journal of the American College of Nutrition* claimed that poor memory could be significantly improved by the intake of foods containing choline. Found in fish, eggs, legumes.

PHENYLALANINE: for brain activity, mood and alertness. Also for headaches, muscle cramps and enhancing production of an appetite suppressant cholycystokinin. Not recommended for diabetes sufferers. Naturally found in fruit, cereals, meat, eggs, bananas.

ARGININE: a vital amino acid that causes the body to release essential hormones. Stimulates sexual maturity, increases lean muscle mass and burns fat, lowers cholesterol, boosts the immune system, speeds recovery from surgery and injury by promoting wound healing. Found in nuts (coconut, pecans, cashews, walnuts, almonds, Brazil nuts, hazel nuts, peanuts), seeds (pumpkin, sesame, sunflower), poultry (chicken and turkey light meat), wild game (pheasant, quail), seafood (halibut, lobster, salmon, shrimp, snails, tuna in water), chickpeas, and cooked soybeans.

ANTIOXIDANTS

Antioxidants attack the free radicals whose harmful chemical reactions can damage the body's cells. It is argued that free-radical damage is the reason we age and, studies have shown, may lead to cancerous cells.

ALPHA LIPOIC ACID: a highly potent antioxidant and immune booster. Helps to protect the liver and pancreas from alcohol damage, ALA also has protective effects on brain and nerve tissue and shows promise as a treatment for stroke and other brain disorders involving free-radical damage. Found in spinach, broccoli and brewer's yeast.

GREEN TEA: reduces high blood pressure, lowers cholestrol. There are four primary polyphenols in green tea: these are powerful antioxidants that have been shown to fight viruses, to slow aging and to have a general beneficial effect on health.

LUTEIN: good for eyes, heart, skin and the reproductive system. Protects against cataract formation. Found in dark-green leafy vegetables, broccoli, cauliflower and Brussels sprouts.

LYCOPENE: said to reduce risk of prostate and lung cancer. Cooked tomatoes are a particularly rich source. Also found in watermelon, guava, pink grapefruit, spinach, peaches and oranges.

ECHINACEA: anti-viral, anti-bacterial and an immune-system stimulant. Good for colds, flu, chronic fatigue and respiratory problems. Derived from the purple coneflower herb.

MILK THISTLE: a purple-flower member of the sunflower family, the seeds of milk thistle have been used by healers for past 2,000 years. Protects the liver and kidney from toxins and pollutants. Good for gall bladder problems, boosting the immune system and may protect against prostate and breast cancer.

ZINC: a mineral comparable to vitamin C, vitamin E, and beta-carotene in antioxidant qualities. Is essential to the growth and function of the reproductive organs; the prostate gland in men contains an abundance of zinc. It is also responsible for regulation of the oil glands, prevention of acne, formation of collagen and bone, wound healing, and a healthy immune system. Food sources include: eggs, kelp, lima beans, pecans and whole grains.

DIGESTIVE AIDS

Digestive aids are herbs and minerals that assist with the digestive process, helping to move food along the digestive pathway. They can also prevent bloating, flatulence and diarrhoea, and help with constipation.

AMYLASE, PEPTIN AND PANCREATIC ENZYMES: supplements needed when the body is producing insufficient amounts of digestive enzymes as a result of impaired liver function or two much acid from food is preventing your own enzymes to work efficiently. Usually available as a complex digestive enzyme.

BROMELAIN: digestive enzyme from fresh pineapple.

CHARCOAL: one of nature's finest absorbent agents. It 'captures', or binds up, unwanted materials and gas then carries it safely through the digestive system. Good for flatulence and diarrhoea.

CHROMIUM: works with *insulin* in assisting cells to take in glucose and release energy. Food sources of chromium are meats, unrefined foods (whole grains, fruits and vegetables), fats and vegetable oils. *Chromium* is a popular supplement for promoting weight loss and stemming food cravings.

GINGER: both fresh or dried improve digestive secretions.

LECITHIN: vital fat emulsifier, stabiliser and antioxidant, contains valuable fatty acid and can be found in soy beans and egg yolk. Is valuable for reducing blood cholesterol levels. Lecithin has been shown to reduce degeneration of the arteries and vital organs, so helping to maintain healthy neural function. Found in soy beans and egg yolk.

PEPPERMINT: an effective remedy to regulate digestion. It has a calming effect on the smooth muscle of the digestive tract and is useful against chills, colic, headaches, indigestion, nausea, IBS and abdominal spasms.

PSYLLIUM HUSK: laxative, high in fibre and viscous lubricants. Psyllium husk comes from the crushed seeds of the *Plantago ovata* plant, an herb native to parts of Asia, Mediterranean regions of Europe, and North Africa. Similar to oats and wheat, psyllium is rich in soluble fibre and is also good for people with high cholesterol. Speeds food along the digestive tract.

SENNA: herbal laxative used for relief of constipation.

ZINC: a mineral that forms part of a powerful antioxidant enzyme essential for the functioning of the immune system. Research suggests that zinc deficiency contributes to the slimming disease *anorexia nervosa* by impairing the sense of taste and smell, and therefore the desire to eat.

LIVER NUTRIENTS

The liver itself has powerful regenerative properties. Up to 60–70 per cent of the liver can actually be destroyed through toxic build up, cancerous growth etc. but then the liver can completely regenerate itself to a full organ.

ANTIOXIDANTS: protective and cleansing, found in fresh raw juices such as carrots, celery, beetroot, dandelions, apples, pears and green drinks such as wheat grass juice, spirulina (a micro algae rich in vegetable protein, beta carotene, iron and vitamin B12).

ESSENTIAL FATTY ACIDS: such as flax seeds (ground and fresh), oily fish, avocado, fresh raw nuts and seeds, cold pressed fresh vegetable oil and seed oil.

LECITHIN: improves the liver's ability to metabolise fats and allows cholesterol to disperse in water so that it can be transported around to the body where it is needed – or eliminated if necessary. It is particularly valuable for those with the condition of a fatty liver for example caused by a poor diet or alcoholism.

METHIONINE: a sulphur-rich amino acid essential for detoxification. Found in legumes, eggs, fish, garlic, onions, seeds and meat.

NATURAL SULPHUR: found in garlic, onions, leeks, shallots, cruciferous vegetables such as broccoli, cauliflower, cabbage and Brussels sprouts.

SELENIUM: a potent antioxidant that detoxifies free radicals. Found in brazil nuts, kelp, brown rice, molasses, seafood, wheat germ, whole grains, garlic and onions.

VITAMIN K: has a critical role in blood clotting and bone nourishment and is found in green leafy vegetables and alfalfa sprouts.

MILK THISTLE: a herb (*Silybum marinum*) found to have remarkable detoxifying and liver-protective effects. It contains a substance called 'silymarin' which protects the liver from severe toxins. For example, there is a poisonous mushroom that can lead to death in 40 per cent of the people who actually ingest it, but taking a milk-thistle extract (or the active ingredient silymarin) can neutralise its affect. It is also one of those herbs prescribed for chronic hepatitis, the inflamed liver condition. Milk thistle is also excellent for improving the functioning of the liver and its regeneration.

KIDNEY MINERALS

Even though my Detox concentrates on cleansing the liver, I do recommend taking supplements that will improve kidney function as well. Like the liver, the kidneys consist of a network of tubules that act as a sieve to eliminate water-soluble toxins from the body. The whole kidney detoxification process works on a very fine mineral balance. The minerals necessary for optimum kidney function are calcium, magnesium, potassium and sodium.

CALCIUM: is vital to the action of every cell in the body. It is also needed to regulate the body's levels of phosphorous, which requires calcium in order to be absorbed into the blood stream; if the body doesn't find enough, it leaches calcium from the bones. Calcium used to be blamed for the formation of calcium kidney stones, but recent research shows that a deficiency of calcium is more likely to be the cause. The richest dietary sources include most dairy products, yogurt, brewer's yeast, Brazil nuts, broccoli, cabbage, dried figs, kelp, dark leafy greens, sardines, soybean flour and tahini.

MAGNESIUM: vital to the kidneys – and every other organ in the body. A deficiency may lead to serious kidney problems. Magnesium activates enzymes, contributes to energy production, and helps regulate the levels of many important nutrients in the body, including calcium and potassium. Like potassium, it is found in nuts, vegetables and fruits – especially bananas.

POTASSIUM: another mineral that helps the kidneys function normally. It acts as a balancing counter-charge to the work of the sodium. Helps the kidneys to excrete more acid. Potassium is widely available in nuts, fruits and vegetables – and also contained in bananas, which is why I recommend them as the only fruit permissible on the detox programme.

SODIUM: the body has to pump sodium salt into the urine to draw water from the blood stream into the kidney tubules. In the process, toxins are transported from the blood to the kidneys for elimination. Diets that are extremely low in salt will impair kidney function.

ADDITIONAL SUPPLEMENTS

The vitamins I would recommend supplementing with are vitamins A, B and C. Vitamin B is especially necessary (particularly for people over 45) because natural sources sometimes contain yeast and phytic acid which can cause digestive disorders. Vitamin B vitamins play a major role in digestion, helping metabolise fats and protein, and in normal functioning of nerves and the nervous system, including keeping our mental functions working. The importance of adequate vitamin B vitamins in the diet cannot be over stressed.

Vegetarians should think about taking extra supplements such as vitamin B12, iron, taurine (vital amino acid) and carnitine (vital amino acid derived from lysine) to avoid poor metabolism and fatigue.

Vegans need to combine three of the following in their diet: grains, nuts, seeds, legumes, other-wise valuable essential amino acids may be deficient. Also soya and tofu make excellent meat and egg substitutes because they are rich in essential amino acids.

Do take care not to overdose on too many vitamins, though. You would do best to take a multivitamin that ensures you are receiving the correct dose of each rather than buying them separately. Taking too many minerals (magnesium, potassium etc) can actually be harmful to the body since they are virtually all metals or metalloids which in large amounts can prove toxic.

A HEALTHY TOXIN-FREE YOU!

My Holistic Diet and Detox Programme is founded on a proper, health-giving, nutritional diet. This alone will have immense benefits – you will lose weight and have far more zest and energy – but it will do far more than that. After your three-week programme, you will have gained a real sense of achievement: finally, you are on the way to being the slimmer, healthier, brighter, more positive person that you have so often imagined yourself to be.

CHAPTER 2
PREPARING TO DETOX

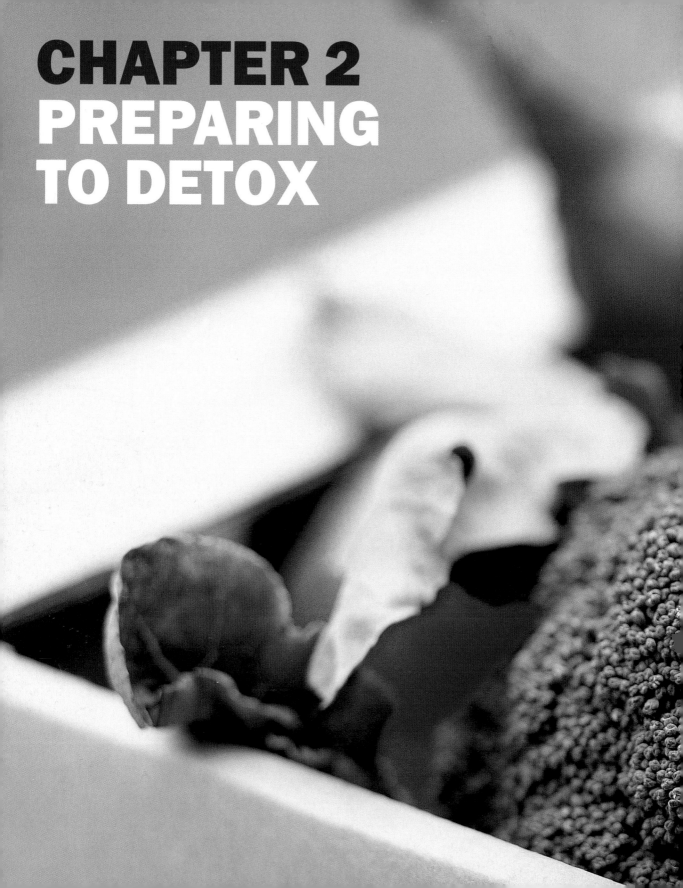

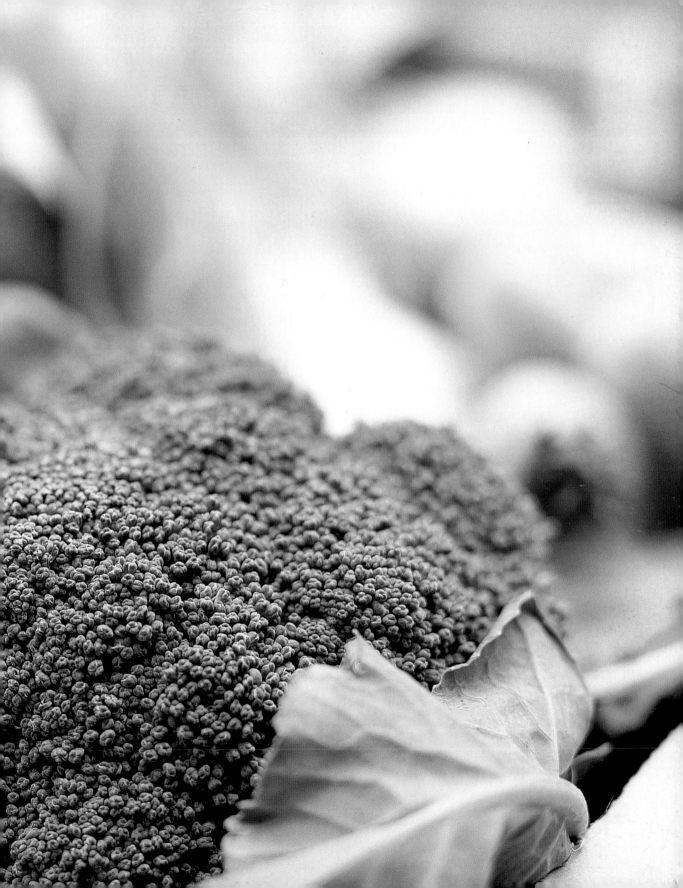

IT IS A MYTH THAT 'DETOX' MEANS COMPLETE SACRIFICE. TO MANY OF US, THE WORD SUGGESTS A PERIOD OF SELF-DENIAL THAT LACKS ANY ENJOYMENT AND DURING WHICH WE MUST DENY OURSELVES ALL THOSE FOODS THAT GIVE US COMFORT AND WHICH WE'VE COME TO RELY ON – NOT JUST FOR TREATS BUT FOR OUR EVERYDAY MEALS.

IT IS TRUE THAT YOU WILL BE ABSTAINING FROM CERTAIN FOODS, SUCH AS WHITE BREAD, PASTA, BISCUITS AND PIZZA, BUT ONLY BECAUSE THEY GIVE RISE TO SYMPTOMS OF INCREASED WEIGHT, LETHARGY, BLOATING, CONSTIPATION, FATIGUE, DEPRESSED IMMUNITY, JOINT ACHES, HEADACHES AND EVEN IMPAIRED MEMORY. IN THEIR PLACE YOU WILL BE DISCOVERING NEW FOODS WHICH NOT ONLY TASTE BETTER (BECAUSE YOUR PALATE WILL BE CLEANER) BUT WHICH WILL ALSO INCREASE YOUR ENERGY LEVELS AND IMPROVE YOUR APPEARANCE AND ENTIRE SENSE OF WELLBEING.

IF YOU WANT YOUR SKIN TO LOOK WONDERFUL, AND IF YOU WANT TO FEEL FULL OF ENERGY AND VITALITY, YOU HAVE TO ENCOURAGE YOURSELF FROM THE INSIDE. ALL OF US LEAD VERY BUSY LIVES, RUSHING AROUND AFTER FAMILIES AND FRIENDS AND MAINTAINING DIFFICULT, DEMANDING JOBS; BUT MY DETOX PROGRAMME IS DESIGNED TO MAKE YOU STOP AND THINK ABOUT YOURSELF, YOUR BODY AND WHAT YOU NEED TO DO TO PROMOTE BETTER HEALTH. TO DO THIS, YOU NEED TO LOOK CLOSELY AT THE NUTRITIONAL VALUE OF THE FOODS YOU EAT AND MAKE THE EFFORT TO PREPARE HEALTHY, WELL-BALANCED MEALS.
   IF, AFTER THE PURIFICATION PROCESS, YOU AUTOMATICALLY START SHOPPING FOR FOODS THAT ARE FAR HEALTHIER, AND START SPENDING MORE TIME ON EATING FRESHLY PREPARED MEALS, THEN YOU WILL FIND THAT THE BENEFITS OF THE DETOX PROGRAMME WILL CONTINUE FOR MANY, MANY, MONTHS – HOPEFULLY, INDEED, FOR THE REST OF YOUR LIFE.

HOW TO SHOP

One of the simplest ways to change your diet is to change the way you shop for food. In Britain, people tend to go to the supermarket once a week and stock up. Everything is then left, for days on end, lying around in the fridge where it loses a lot of its nutritional content. I prefer the European approach where people shop on a daily basis for their provisions, be it from the market or the fishmonger or a local grocer.

Although it may not be possible to buy food every day, try to shop on a much more regular basis – maybe two or three times a week. If possible, visit a farmers' market at the weekend and, during the week, purchase fresh produce from local retailers or the supermarket. Get just enough vegetables for that day and maybe the next day. Buy some fresh fish or, if you're not going to eat the whole chicken, get a chicken portion instead. This will be hugely beneficial to your diet because, the fresher the food, the more nutrients you can derive from it.

JUNKING THE JUNK FOOD

Did you know that burgers, chips, chocolate, biscuits and sweets aren't good for you? Of course you did. High in fats, sugars and additives, they provide very little nutritional content and also lead to rapid weight gain. But did you know that ready-made meals may be just as bad? The United Kingdom is now the highest consumer of pre-packaged meals in Europe: one-third of us now have supermarket meals more than once a week. While this may be convenient, they fail to provide us with anything like the necessary amounts of energy or nutrients.

This 'food' is pumped full of salt and preservatives so that it can be stored for longer. It is given artificial flavourings to 'improve' its taste, and starch, a thickening and bulking agent, to improve its appearance. Then, almost to add insult to injury, these products are packaged in plastic so that, when we heat them up in the microwave or the oven, the chemicals from the containers will leak into the food.

These ready meals deposit, in your system, chemicals and toxic waste that stop the body from functioning at the proper level – making you feel tired, below par, and generally unwell. The next thing, once you've broken the weekly shop habit, that I suggest you do when you're assessing the way you shop is, therefore, rethink your journey around the different aisles in the supermarket. Avoid the sections full of processed meals and head, instead, for the fresh fruit and vegetables, the fresh chickens and the fish counter.

Opting for this type of produce requires a bit more commitment and effort, but such foods will prove to be much more nutritious, better value for money and less harmful to your body. As part of the Holistic Programme, you should be investing more time in yourself. If that means spending 20 minutes a day grilling chicken or steaming fish with vegetables, it is time well invested. Such food is far better for you than a reduced-fat, pre-packaged lasagne that is full of chemicals and, in all likelihood, will leave you feeling hungry and dissatisfied.

RICHARD'S STORY

It had been a very difficult year and I was feeling extremely tired. I went away for Christmas and had a good rest but, when I came back, I just didn't feel refreshed or re-energised. I was also very overweight. My girlfriend persuaded me to see Joshi. I decided to go and have a chat. I thought he might be able to help me with my diet because I am a vegetarian who doesn't eat fish. I ate what I thought was a healthy diet, no processed or fried foods, but when I went to see him he just looked at me in horror.

He could see I was very overweight and said I needed to detox. He gave me a blood test and then introduced me to this new way of eating. I loved fruit but he cut that out of my diet, and then he cut out certain vegetables that I really enjoyed such as mushrooms, cucumber, tomatoes, aubergines and courgettes – because they are acidic, or members of the nightshade family. I didn't eat much dairy produce, but I wasn't allowed that either, nor bread or wheat products. He told me I had to start eating fish, as I wasn't getting sufficient protein. I hadn't eaten fish for twenty years – but it wasn't a problem, and now I eat it every day.

The effect of going on the Detox was almost immediate. I felt better within a couple of days. Even though I had been eating what I thought were healthy foods, I ate too much and did no exercise. I had been on some kind of diet most of my life but nothing ever worked. However, with Joshi's Detox I could feel the weight falling off me. I have never been into weighing myself, but I lost about 10 inches around my waist. I wasn't so tired, I was sleeping much better and, within a couple of weeks, people were saying how well I looked. My skin had a better colour and I was losing the weight.

The hardest thing was giving up fruit, which I know is very acidic, but I loved it. I never used to drink very much but, on the Detox, I could drink vodka (neat), which suited me.

I found Joshi inspirational. Not only did he get me to eat fish, but to join a gym, which I never dreamed I would do. I always regarded personal trainers as akin to the devil! But I did join a gym and, even though I travel quite a lot, I work out every day that I'm in London. I suppose I stuck 100 per cent to the Detox Diet for about a year, and now I still stick to it 90 per cent of the time (I do have the odd slice of bread). I have also had colonic irrigation, which is fantastic. I feel so well.

Initially your body goes into positive shock, and you feel a bit light-headed, but then everything settles down and it is quite easy. I just feel so much better eating this way that I don't see the point of changing.

RICHARD DAVIES, 53, IS CHAIRMAN OF A RECORD COMPANY AND LIVES IN LONDON.

HOW FRESH IS OUR FOOD?

The length of time for which supposedly fresh produce can now be stored is truly shocking. The apples and potatoes on the supermarket shelves may have been sitting in cold storage for up to a year. Carrots, which are often cooled in chlorinated water before packing, can be stored for anything from five to nine months, and even products with a much shorter shelf life are filled with chemicals to make them last just a few days longer.

Lettuce is now preserved using a process called 'modified-atmosphere packaging' (map). Salad leaves for the popular mixed bags are dried and sorted before being packaged in pillows of plastic. Here, the normal levels of oxygen and carbon dioxide have been altered to slow any visible deterioration or discolouring. The leaves are then treated with a chlorine-based compound, an antioxidant or a preservative, to keep them looking fresh for up to ten days.

Bananas are picked in the Caribbean when they are bullet hard and bright green so that they can be kept for up to two weeks. They are loaded into warehouses where ethylene gas is discharged from cylinders or cartridges, catalysing the hormonal process of ripening.

Most UK tomatoes and cucumbers are now grown hydroponically – without soil. The plants are rooted in rockwool (similar to roofing insulation), and a computer-controlled irrigation system adds essential nutrients and water. There are, in fact, some benefits to this: because the environment is so controlled, farmers can use far less pesticides. However, the levels of nutrients in the produce are severely depleted.

Like bananas, lots of tomatoes are picked when they are green and allowed to ripen in warehouses or even on supermarket shelves. You may be tempted to choose them because you think – quite rightly – that they will last longer when we get them home, but it also means they won't have any nutritional value. All foods need sunlight to synthesise their nutrients so, if the produce is unripe when it is picked, the nutritional content will be negligible and it will effectively be hollow, Hence the importance of picking fruit which has been vine-ripened. It is a question of quality, not quantity: three ripe tomatoes will provide more vitamins than twenty which have been pre-packed after possibly being picked six weeks before ripening.

You also need to commit to eating produce as close as possible to the time it has been picked. Cutting and harvesting fruit and vegetables exposes them to air or sunlight and leaves them vulnerable to the ongoing process of oxidation (when oxygen and certain chemicals combine to change cell structure). When this happens, their nutritional value becomes depleted; so, for instance, after fresh vegetables are cut up and turned into prepared packs, their vitamin C level drops markedly.

Therefore, frozen can sometimes be a better option. Vegetables retain a lot of their nutrients when they are frozen immediately after picking. Similarly, frozen fish is often packed in trays of ice just hours after it has been caught, and so valuable minerals and vitamins are not lost. I do not, however, advise using frozen chickens because they are often packed with chemicals and water to keep them hydrated for longer.

USE-BY, SELL-BY, AND BEST-BEFORE DATES

There is a confusing variety of dates and instructions on our foods today. Food that is highly perishable and that can cause food poisoning (such as poultry, meat, fish and some dairy products) has a use-by date. Never eat any food or drink after its use-by date, even if it looks and smells fine. Foods that can safely be kept for some time, such as canned and frozen foods, aren't given use-by dates but the less-prescriptive best-before dates. Although they are unlikely to be harmful if eaten soon after that, they will have lost a lot of their nutritional value.

The classification I find most useful is the sell-by or display-until date. This is used by the shop to show how quickly that item must be bought by the public. I recommend that, when buying foods in a supermarket, you eat them by the sell-by date because they will still be fairly fresh and have a higher concentration of nutrients.

Best of all, certainly when buying fruit and vegetables, is to opt for produce that is loose, rather than pre-packaged – which won't have any instructions on it at all. This is less likely to have been treated to prolong its shelf life. You will instinctively pick out the loose items that look the freshest, using common sense rather than a label to guide you.

BUYING THE BEST YOU CAN AFFORD

You don't necessarily have to buy the most expensive food, but it is important to buy food that is as fresh and as chemical free as possible. Industrial farming has resulted in cheap, mass-produced foods that frequently lack the nutrients and vitamins your body needs – and can be full of toxins. Low-cost chickens and turkeys, for instance, will have been injected with growth hormones and pumped full of water and starch, as well as being laden with chemicals.

It's true that food that has not been intensively farmed does cost more. However, I firmly believe that it's simply a matter of reordering our priorities. I find it incredible that people begrudge paying for good, healthy, nutritious food but think nothing of spending hundreds of pounds on the artificial things in life, such as the latest designer trainers or a Plasma TV screen. If we spend just a small proportion more on a better-quality diet, we will be buying a healthier body, an increasingly attractive appearance and more energy – a better quality of life.

IS ORGANIC BETTER?

There is a lot of debate as to whether organic produce is really healthier than that grown using conventional methods. As I've mentioned, organic isn't always better; it depends on where the food has been produced and how.

The Soil Association, Britain's leading organic organisation and voluntary regulator, has stringent criteria. It stipulates that organic food: 'avoids the use of artificial chemical fertilisers and pesticides on the land, relying instead on developing a healthy fertile soil and growing a mixture of crops.' The organic symbol is a reliable guide that the produce is certified to high organic standards.

However, over 70 per cent of the organic food that is sold in Britain is imported and standards do vary from country to country. Furthermore, there are many things about which no country can lay down rules. It is impossible, for instance, to control the movement of the clouds and the quality of the water they contain or the levels of pollutants in the atmosphere. Nor is it possible to control the nutritional content of the soil itself. One agricultural society produced a paper, a few years ago, stating that almost 30 per cent of the agricultural soil in England was devoid of any nutritional content at all.

In terms of fruit and vegetables, the best course of action is to look at the different produce and see how it looks and feels. Most importantly, it must be ripe. If the organic produce in the local supermarket looks healthy and the colours are bright and it is ready to eat, then that is the best option. If, however, the fruit and vegetables haven't ripened sufficiently, or if they look bruised or wrinkly, I would suggest opting for standard produce that is in season. It is more likely to have been locally and naturally produced and so contain a higher level of nutrients.

In terms of fish and white meats such as chicken and turkey, organic is definitely better. The flesh may be a bit leaner but at least it will be free of the chemicals, pesticides and hormones that will have been inflicted on the non-organic varieties.

I once went to a very interesting Christmas lunch at the house of the Deputy British High Commissioner in Calcutta. The Norfolk turkey that had been sent over from England was a substantial size – enough for about twenty people. The Commissioner had also been sent, as gifts from the other countries represented there, turkeys – which were of a similar size. Then, he showed me the turkey that had arrived from the American Embassy. It was enormous, the size of a small cow. It must have been genetically modified. Its carcass, grossly distorted by growth hormone injections, was probably also crammed full of toxins.

This might explain why, in America, obesity is one of the fastest-growing diseases in the world. Obesity, 'the deposition of fat and the slowing down of one's metabolism' is related to the amount of toxins that we have within our bodies. On the whole, therefore, organic foods are preferable but with the proviso that we look carefully at the different fruit and vegetables for sale before we buy them.

WHAT ABOUT BIODYNAMIC FARMING?

Although biodynamic farming is the oldest non-chemical agricultural movement, predating organic farming by over twenty years, it is still something of a new trend in the consumer world.

Biodynamic farming is a holistic style of agriculture in which the mineral, plant, animal and human kingdoms work in harmony to produce nutritious food and regenerate the soil in tune with the natural rhythms of the moon, the planets and the stars. These solar bodies influence the optimum times to sow, cultivate and harvest the crops.

The biodynamic system considers the farm as a self-contained, self-regulating unit. Emphasis is placed on the integration of animals and plants, similar perhaps to our childhood vision of farms as distinct from the current monocultures that exist today.

Ideally, animals are born on the farm and fed with produce grown on the farm's land, which has been fertilised with their manure. Developed from a series of lectures given by Austrian philosopher Rudolf Steiner, it is a system that thrives on diversity and, in common with good organic practice, plenty of rotation.

One important element of this system is biodynamic composting. This is a complex and scientific way of recycling animal and plant waste materials for the benefit of the soil, the animals, the plants and the farm itself. A study at Washington State University found that the preparations used in biodynamic composting have a significant effect on the composting process whereby it matures faster and is richer in nitrates than compost created by conventional methods.

The end result of all of these processes is to produce food, be it plant or animal based, that is rich in life forces that create optimum nutrition. It also tastes better and does no harm to the environment during its production.

There are biodynamic farms and gardens in more than 30 countries on five continents. Biodynamic produce is marketed under the Demeter symbol and there is an International Demeter network co-ordinating the work of Demeter organisations worldwide.

PAUL'S STORY

I was recommended to see Joshi by a friend. I was very fat and determined not to be fat by the time I got to my fortieth birthday. I had tried lots of diets but nothing had worked. My diet was not good. Most of the time I would eat sandwiches and jacket potatoes for lunch, or eat out. My job entails a lot of entertaining and eating out late. I often would have quick café meals at lunchtime and then cakes and biscuits mid-afternoon.

However, I found the detox surprisingly easy to follow. I did it quite strictly for seven months! I had a lot of weight to lose. Initially I didn't think there was anything I could eat; but then I realised that, if I ate freshly prepared meals, I could eat lots of things. The other reason for embarking on the Detox was because I had no energy. I felt very lethargic and I needed rejuvenating. I also had a nasty skin infection that wouldn't go away. Within about four weeks, I really noticed a change. I felt more alert and healthier. I had replaced my intake of coffee and tea with peppermint tea. I drank lots more water and cut out snacking on cakes and biscuits – and also fruit. I was never a big drinker, so absence of alcohol wasn't a problem. I cut out all sugar and wheat and this made a huge difference. In fact, when I did have sugar, I immediately felt bloated. I had no red meat. Strangely, the food I missed most was mushrooms!

As I re-educated my palate, I did not crave sweet things. In fact, when I did have some grapes I found them too sweet. I had lost one and half stone in six weeks and two and a half stone by my fortieth birthday in April. I found wheat-free bread, or bread made with spelt flour, very useful as snacks. I also developed a taste for natural yoghurt, which I never liked before. People started commenting on my weight loss and improved complexion, and I started to feel brave enough to go to the gym. I also started to have breakfast, which I never used to do and which sustained me through to lunch (by which time I only needed a small meal). Gluten-free cornflakes with rice milk and a banana, which was fantastic, was my daily breakfast staple.

I found the supplements a huge benefit. Whether that was just psychological, or whether they did help to kick start me, I don't care – they worked. Even though I have been off the Detox Programme for a while, now, I have stuck to the foods Joshi recommends. Even with a bit of cheating, I haven't put on any weight.

If I go out for meals with friends, I can usually find something on a menu that suits. French restaurants are best because you can order something straightforward such as grilled chicken or fish with vegetables. Joshi is very realistic in that he knows that if you go on holiday, or spend a weekend away, you will cheat – and that is okay. As he tells you, his Detox is about cutting down on foods rather than cutting out; although for me, cutting out has been easier than I ever expected.

PAUL SPYKER, 40, IS A THEATRICAL AGENT AND PRODUCER.

GENETICALLY MODIFIED FOOD

Despite consumers' opposition to genetically modified foods, they have infiltrated the food chain. So, unless you are buying organic produce that is free from GM material, your food will probably contain some GM derivative. This is despite fears of unknown long-term health risks and an unleashing of new toxins and allergens which could have untold effects on ourselves and our environment.

A genetically modified plant is one that is changed so that it produces certain characteristics and is resistant to insects and weed killers. The main foods produced this way include soybean, oilseed rape and maize. Presently, GM crops are not yet grown in this country but the UK government has given the go-ahead for the production of genetically modified maize.

GM foods have to be labelled – with the exception of those that contain small amounts, namely 0.9 per cent or less. According to the United States Food Standards Agency, however, labelling is scant at best and, for most processed foods, merely declares that they contain some GM material. According to a *Which?* Report, published in September 2004, supermarkets such as Asda, Budgens, Coop, Iceland, Morrisons, Marks & Spencer, Somerfield, Sainsbury's, Tesco and Waitrose all try to avoid GM ingredients in their own-brand products but cannot guarantee that the animals who end up on the meat counter are not fed GM feed. The law that requires GM foods to be labelled also requires that restaurants should declare if any of their food contains GM elements – but few know whether they do or not. The jury is still out on the long-term affects of GM crops. However, what is certain is that their nutritional composition will inevitably be altered and, for the moment, we don't know whether that will be for better or worse.

YOUR IDEAL SHOPPING BASKET

It is time to ditch everything that you have in your store cupboards and start again. Out go the pasta, white bread and sugary breakfast cereals that sap all your energy, and in come the nutritious fresh alternatives.

The first things to add to your shopping basket are some bottles of still mineral water (glass bottles are preferable to plastic) or, even better, a water filter. This will provide you with a clean supply of bacteria-free tap water and – as water is essential to cleanse, hydrate and purify your system – the purer the water, the cleaner the insides of your body.

Starting with breakfast, you will need plain bio yoghurt (which is usually made from cow's milk but, in small amounts, that's OK) or, if you are lactose intolerant, soya or rice yoghurt. To go with it, add honey and organic bananas.

Instead of Coco Pops or Cornflakes, buy gluten-free/yeast-free muesli and rice or soya milk (vanilla is a flavour option, for a change). If you can't go without your slice of toast in the morning, then make it with a wheat-free rye bread (look in your supermarket for the new gluten-free/yeast-free brands). Instead of butter, use an olive-oil or a pumpkin spread. A deliciously healthy alternative would be an organic poached egg.

Next into the basket will be the ingredients for lunch and dinner. Buy some fresh lettuce (preferably not the bagged variety), asparagus, spinach, broccoli, cabbage, bok choi and mange tout. You can use these in salads – or steam or stir-fry them, so make sure you have a wok or a large frying pan and a steamer. Onions, shallots, and garlic are all wonderful vegetables that should be used generously as they allow your liver to detox, thanks to the special enzymes and minerals they contain. As a back-up, frozen mixed vegetables are not only useful for curries and stews but they will be on hand in a last-minute crisis. Furthermore, they are a valuable source of nutrients because vegetables for freezing are often picked and frozen while still fresh.

For protein, buy fresh chicken breasts (preferably organic and thus not full of water) and fresh fish such as salmon, haddock or halibut. For carbohydrates, you need brown rice and brown-rice pasta or brown-rice noodles. Brown rice is more fibrous on the gut wall and so helps clean it. White rice, on the other hand, tends to be more gluey and has had most of its nutritional content removed. If you are a vegetarian, or are going to be cooking vegetarian meals, then you'll need soya or tofu pieces to provide all your necessary non-meat proteins.

I, personally, advocate steaming or grilling fish, chicken, and vegetables. However, a little oil is still needed for such methods, or for salad dressings, so buy the best-quality extra-virgin olive oil that you can afford because it contains far fewer chemicals than a lot of the cheaper, processed varieties. For stir-fries, however, I recommend sesame oil or sunflower oil, which are both very good for reducing cholesterol levels.

It is a combination of low blood-sugar levels and the release of small amounts of gastric juice that make people feel hungry. My Detox Programme shows you how to control both these factors so that you won't feel the usual overwhelming urge for chocolate or crisps during the day. However, in case you do feel like a snack, make sure you have on hand some rice cakes, gluten-free oatcakes, hummus, chopped carrots, cauliflower and mange-tout. Try, if possible, to make your own hummus from tinned or dried

chickpeas and guacamole (see Recipes chapter) because the shop-bought versions are full of vinegar, sugar and additives. To eat with the hummus, get organic celery and carrots which you can chop into sticks and also nibble, just by themselves, as a healthy snack alternative, thereby helping to level out any changes in your blood sugar.

For flavouring, I favour naturally derived rock salt or sea salt. Low-sodium salt is chemically synthesised and so it isn't necessarily better for us. And always have a supply of fresh herbs – such as mint, coriander, dill, thyme and rosemary – on hand. These can add immeasurably to salads and can also be used as a marinade for fish or chicken.

For dessert, some live bio yoghurt or soya yoghurt with a teaspoon of honey is delicious; or think about trying some gluten-free/yeast-free and sugar-free biscuits. They're made from spelt flour, honey or molasses, desiccated coconut and rice milk and are available from good health food shops. In place of coffee and black tea, add lots of herbal teas (peppermint, camomile, fenugreek etc.) and green teas, to your shopping basket – take a look in the local health-food store to see the incredible variety of different alternatives. If you think you can't live without coffee, there is a caffeine-free, chicory-oats alternative that tastes like coffee but is much better for you. Similarly, two tea substitutes called Wake Up and Two Char are very good because they don't contain the dyes and tannins found in normal tea or coffee. If you need a sweetener in your tea or coffee, then rice syrup, molasses or honey is a good alternative to sugar, although honey, in vast quantities, can be slightly acidic.

Fresh vegetable juices are an invaluable addition to your diet and for these you will need fresh beetroot, celery, spinach, wheatgrass, carrots and radishes. I also recommend adding fresh mint and ginger to all your juices to give them an extra fresh and zesty zing. If you have a blender, you can make smoothies using either soya yoghurt or a live bio yoghurt. Add some chopped banana or some chopped almonds, a little bit of cardamom to taste, if you like, and a drizzle of honey. This also makes a lovely snack or dessert alternative. (For more information about juices and juicing, see Chapter 4.)

Note: All statistics for percentages of organic food sold taken from a Soil Association Survey carried out from 15 November to 15 December 2003

SUPERMARKET SHOPPING

Getting out of the supermarkets and into local shops and farmers' markets is a really good idea, but sometimes we all need to use a supermarket. All the major UK supermarket chains now carry ranges of organic food plus wheat-free, gluten-free and dairy free lines. Thanks to consumer pressure, they now try to source more of their fresh produce from the UK. As at September 2004, 70 per cent of organic food (on average) was imported. The Government has set a target to invert the balance so that 70 per cent of organic food on sale in supermarkets will be sourced from the UK by 2010. None of the supermarkets is either consistently good or consistently bad. Whichever shop you are in, look for foods that are fresh and ripe and, therefore, bursting with vitamins and minerals.

Marks & Spencer

Unlike most major food retailers in the UK and Ireland, Marks & Spencer only sells 'own label' products. It has a much smaller organic range (approximately 400 products) than some of the larger supermarkets but the quality of all their produce tends to be high. M&S do not use food irradiation (a process used by many other supermarkets, which exposes food to a carefully controlled amount of ionising energy in order to kill micro-organisms such as salmonella and E.coli, thus lengthening the food's shelf-life). They also run Select Farms, their own farm assurance scheme, which employs specially trained auditors to guarantee high levels in food production.

M&S also source a lot of their produce from the UK. According to a Soil Association survey in 2003, 95 per cent of their organic chickens are UK sourced plus 100 per cent of their organic carrots but only 58 per cent of their organic potatoes. The best thing to do, when shopping in M&S, is keep an eye out for their 'Best of Season' range which lets you know when certain crops are at their optimum in terms of their natural and traditional season.

Sainsbury's

Sainsbury's has been selling organic food since 1986 and their range now extends to more than 1,300 lines, from bread to baby foods. The supermarket currently imports 60 per cent of its organic food range. In 2004, the supermarket was in the process of dropping the import ratio of its organic food range from 60 per cent to 45 per cent. In the Soil Association Survey, 93 per cent of its organic chickens, 95 per cent of its organic potatoes and 96 per cent of its organic carrots were sourced in the UK. They sell, in different shops throughout the country, over 3,500 local or regional products.

Sainsbury's was the first store to introduce a range of gluten-free/wheat-free and dairy-free products called 'Free From', in 2002. They still have one of the best ranges for sufferers from any grain or dairy allergies. They also have a very good health-foods section that offers a wide range of different products that are free from artificial flavours, colours, sweeteners and preservatives. These products contain no genetically modified organisms or derivatives and have limited amounts of hydrogenated fat and refined sugars.

Waitrose

In 1983, Waitrose became one of the first supermarkets to start selling organic produce. Back then, only one per cent of all the fruit and vegetables sold was organic. That figure has now risen to 12 per cent. Some 60 per cent of the chain's baby food is organic and they stock over 1,300 organic product lines.

The supermarket's commitment to organic produce is genuine. They were one of the first companies to sign up to the Organic Targets Bill which aims to ensure that 30 per cent of our farmland is organic by 2010. They also work closely with UK farmers in a bid to source more organic produce from this country; this has the extra benefit of cutting down on the distances that organic food has to travel. The 2003 Soil Association survey that found that 100 per cent of Waitrose's organic chicken, 100 per cent of their organic carrots and 99 per cent of their organic potatoes were sourced from the UK.

They also stock an impressive array of gluten-free/wheat-free breads as well as a healthy number of dairy-free ranges.

Asda

Asda says that it buys British 'wherever possible'. In the 2003 Soil Association survey, 96 per cent of its organic carrots, 87 per cent of chickens and 74 per cent of potatoes were locally sourced. The supermarket now sources 100 per cent of its fresh turkey and chicken from the UK and in 2005 expects 100 per cent of the carrots stocked to be from British farms. Asda has also worked with farmers to extend the British carrot-growing season from 46 to 49 weeks and the British season for new, baby and salad potatoes by 10 weeks. In the past, it had to start importing these ranges in November; now British stock is on the shelves until January.

Although the supermarket does stock organic lines and a small number of gluten-free/wheat-free and dairy-free products, this is still on a relatively small scale in comparison to the other supermarkets.

BOX SCHEMES

Home delivery box schemes are an excellent way of ensuring a constant supply of fresh, in-season, locally grown, organic produce. If you need to know about box schemes in your area, you can check your local paper, or contact The Soil Association, or log on to www.alotoforganics.co.uk. Suppliers such as London-based Abel and Cole, organic retailer of the year 2004, work in partnership with UK growers and producers to supply – packed in recyclable packaging – meat, fish, fruit and vegetables. Over 70 per cent of the produce is grown locally.

FARMERS' MARKETS

Farmers' markets have grown in popularity partly because the farmer is usually there, selling his produce direct to the public, and available to answer questions. All the products must be grown, reared, caught, brewed, pickled, baked, smoked or processed by whoever is the stallholder, and comply with regulations laid down by FARMA standards. You can be assured that everything you buy at a farmers market has been home grown. (See Directory section for information on farmers markets.)

STORING AND PREPARING FOOD

Try not to store too much food, be it fresh, frozen or already cooked. I particularly don't favour eating leftovers from the day before because they are not fresh and have lost much of their nutritional content. A proportion of the food's goodness was lost during the cooking process and then further destroyed by coming into contact with the air where it has become slowly oxidised and broken down.

You can freeze fresh fruit and vegetables but make sure they are left whole rather than chopped so that the nutritional blanket which envelopes them remains intact. Most food should be frozen raw, although blanching is also effective: because it kills the food's resident microbes, this will then remain healthy for a few days longer. However, I tend not to freeze any food for more than five to ten days so that all the minerals and vitamins are still active when it's eaten.

If you have a family and they are not joining you on the Detox Programme, it helps, psychologically, to have a separate shelf in the fridge and the cupboard for your Detox Programme food. In this way, all the provisions for the rest of the family, such as butter, milk products, sugary cereals, coffees and teas, are not there to cause temptation when you are most vulnerable. But don't feel you have to avoid the family altogether; I will show how you can integrate your menus with those of other members in your household and get everyone eating healthier food.

One final note on a key point: I cannot overstate the importance of washing all fruit and vegetables before you use them, to make sure that they have been thoroughly cleansed of all chemical residues left over from the farming process. The World Health Organisation (WHO) has listed over two thousand known pesticides that are used around the world to stop insects from destroying crops. Most of these will find their way into the supermarket – on food. The Soil Association reports that in the UK alone, around 25,000 tonnes of pesticide are applied to crops every year and 350 chemicals are routinely used in British conventional farming. A Cox's apple, for instance, may have been sprayed 16 times with 36 different chemicals. All these toxic chemicals, therefore, need to be cleaned from your food before you eat it.

A DIFFERENT WAY OF EATING

It is, of course, not just what we eat but how we eat that is important. The recipes for the Detox Programme will look at different ways of preparing meals. They will show you how to steam, grill, and poach foods in ways that will enhance all the flavour without adding any extra fat or flavourings that would upset the body's natural pH balance. And of course, a fundamental part of this programme is about taking a little time to prepare meals, lovingly, for yourself.

CHAPTER 3
DETOX FOODS

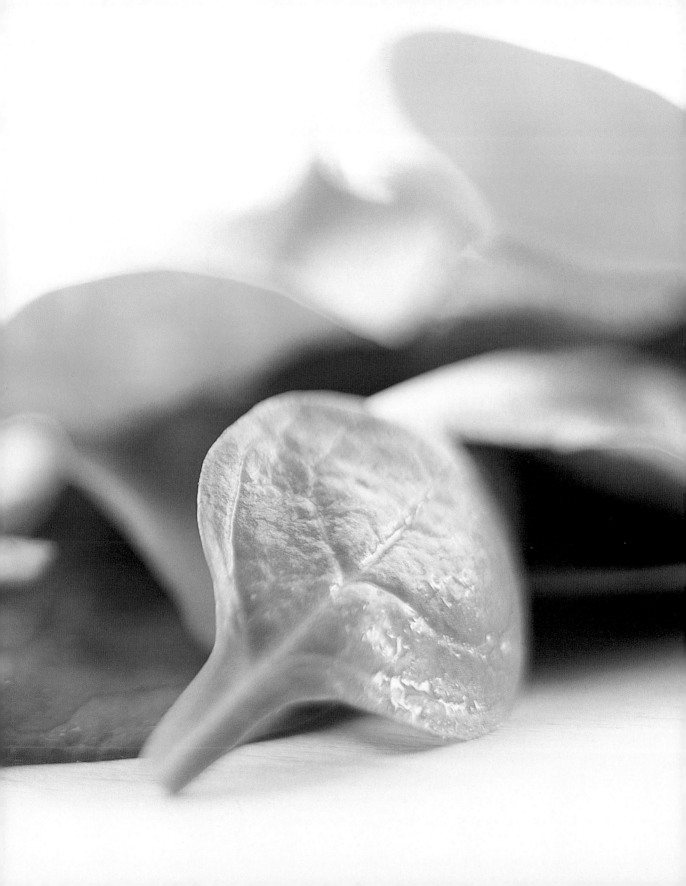

YOU NOW HAVE A GOOD IDEA OF ALL THE WORK YOUR LIVER HAS TO DO TO OFFSET THE DAMAGING EFFECTS OF TOXINS THAT FIND THEIR WAY INTO YOUR BODY. YOU'RE ALSO AWARE OF THE ADDITIONAL BURDEN IT BEARS BECAUSE OF THE TREMENDOUS BIAS IN MOST WESTERN DIETS TOWARDS ACIDIC FOODS, AND THE STRAIN (THROUGH THEIR TOXIC WASTES AND THE LACK OF NOURISHMENT THAT THEY OFFER) THEY PUT ON YOUR WHOLE SYSTEM. THIS CHAPTER IS ABOUT REDRESSING THIS ACID IMBALANCE AND MOVING FIRMLY BACK INTO ALKALINE TERRITORY.

THE FOOD PROGRAMME THAT YOU ARE ABOUT TO FOLLOW IS NOT AN ALKALINE DIET. IT IS A HOLISTIC METABOLIC DETOX THAT IS DESIGNED TO IMPROVE THE FUNCTIONING OF YOUR ORGANS AND YOUR BODY'S METABOLISM. BUT BECAUSE YOU UNDOUBTEDLY CONSUME TOO MANY ACIDIC FOODS (EVERYBODY DOES), YOU NEED TO CUT THE ACID RIGHT BACK AND INCREASE THE ALKALINE SO THAT 70–75 PER CENT OF WHAT GOES INTO YOUR MOUTH IS ALKALINE OR ALKALINE-FORMING.

TOP TEN DETOX RULES

- **NO RED MEAT**
- **NO DAIRY PRODUCE**
- **NO FRUIT – EXCEPT BANANAS**
- **NO WHEAT, GLUTEN, YEAST**
- **NO ALCOHOL**
- **NO BISCUITS, CAKES, DOUGHNUTS**
- **NO JAMS, SPREADS – EXCEPT HONEY**
- **NO COFFEE, DECAFFEINATED COFFEE OR TEA – EXCEPT HERBAL TEAS**
- **NO SUGAR, CHOCOLATE OR SWEETS**
- **NO ARTIFICIALLY PRODUCED FLAVOURINGS: TOMATO KETCHUP, VINEGAR, MUSTARD ETC.**

SALIVA PH TEST

The concentration of acidity or alkalinity in a solution is denoted by a figure known as 'pH' that works on a scale of 1–14.

Anything less than 7 is acidic, 7 is neutral, and above 7 is alkaline. Your desired balance is a slightly alkaline 7.3 or 7.4.

You can test your own acid/alkaline balance using your saliva and pH paper (also called litmus paper) which is available from most chemists.

This is a simple test that will show you whether you have a higher than normal concentration of acid in your body and, therefore, an increased susceptibility to various aliments and diseases.

→ First of all, wait at least two hours after eating.
→ Fill your mouth with saliva and then swallow it.
→ Repeat this step to help ensure that your saliva is clean.
→ The third time, put some of your saliva onto the pH paper.
→ The pH paper should turn blue. If it is blue, this indicates that your saliva is slightly alkaline at a healthy pH of 7.4.

If the pH paper does not turn blue, compare the colour you get with the chart that comes with the pH paper and see how acidic you've become.

After the first week of the three-week Detox, check and see whether you are becoming 'any bluer'. By the end of the third week, you should certainly see a difference.

If you follow my advice for three weeks, so drastic are the effects of this re-balancing exercise that you may no longer need certain prescription medications because your elevated blood pressure and cholesterol levels will have both dropped. (Do consult your doctor about altering any prescription medicines though.) Your body will be cleansed and in balance. For this reason, I advise my patients to avoid most fruits, even those that are alkaline, to allow the body to burn more fat and hence release more toxins.

My Holistic Detox is not just about getting rid of acidic foods, though, but about improving your overall health and vitality. In order to achieve this, I am crossing certain alkaline foods off your Detox Diet list as well. Where these are fruits or vegetables, it means I am eliminating them because they are often picked before they've ripened when they still contain too much acid and sugar. Other alkaline foods are being banished because I consider them to be nutritionally hollow.

I shall, however, include some foods that are slightly acidic – eggs, for example. Egg white is alkaline but the egg yolk is acidic. Egg yolks are included in the Detox Programme because they are a valuable source of the proteins and amino acids that are necessary for liver detoxification.

ALKALINE CAN BE ACID-FORMING!

There are two types of acid and alkaline foods. The first are those that actually contain acids or alkalis (soluble salts). The second group consists of acid- or alkaline-*forming* foods. This term refers to what happens after these foods have been combined with digestive juices in the body. In all natural foods, both of these elements are present but one is stronger. It is the alkaline-forming foods that are most relevant to the job of changing the body's pH to its slightly alkaline 'neutral'. Acidic food causes acidity to flow into the muscles. This results in mineral salts being deposited – calcium, for example (taken from our bones) – because their job is to neutralise the acid. The combination of acid and mineral salts, however, leads to increased tightening of the muscle and a constriction of the blood flow. This, in turn, leads to a build up of lactic acid, dead cells and debris that cannot be filtered. These toxins are stored in fat cells that may then 'morph' into the subcutaneous fat known as cellulite. As you know, my Detox is more often about cutting down than cutting out. You will be reducing the number of acid-forming foods you eat but not cutting them all out because they may not necessarily be acidic all of the time. A lemon, for example, which is a very acid fruit, turns alkaline when combined with the juices and digestive acids already present in the body. It is important to bear this principle in mind when referring to the Acid/Alkaline Food Chart, which labels the foods according to the effect they have on the body.

FOOD INTOLERANCES

The intention of this Detox programme is not only to introduce as many alkalising foods as possible so as to reduce the body's acidity (which is vitally important for detoxification), but also to reduce a lot of foods to which we have, over the years, developed an intolerance.

Food intolerance is the body's inability either to digest or process certain foods or chemicals contained within those foods. As distinct from a food allergy, which is an immune reaction, intolerance manifests itself in symptoms such as bloating, indigestion, wind, stomach pain or diarrhoea.

Allergy reactions tend to be more acute: a rash, difficulty in breathing, swollen eyes and lips, a runny nose or headaches. They can also be more debilitating – migraines, for example, which are not-uncommon reactions to caffeine and chocolate. The body usually develops an immune/intolerance reaction to acidic foods such as tomatoes, sugar, dairy produce, wheat, shellfish, nuts, chocolate and coffee.

You can, however, develop an intolerance to a protein in milk, for instance, while having no reaction to eating butter and cheese. I have an intolerance to eating fruit in this country – but not when I am in India. I think this is because the fruit is picked when it is ripe in India – but not here.

Most people can endure food tolerances. They may be all right most of the time and then suddenly find they feel uncomfortable or bloated after eating a particular food. However, if not heeded, intolerances can turn into full-blown allergies. It is well worth, therefore, being aware of foods to which you're intolerant so that you don't overeat them.

ALKALINE-FORMING AND ACID-FORMING FOODS

FOODS IN RED ARE:

Acid-forming in the human body

Make blood, lymph and saliva more acid and

Cause acidosis – too much acid in the body

(lower pH number)

FOODS IN BLUE ARE:

Alkaline-forming in the human body

Make blood, lymph and saliva more alkaline

and Cause alkalosis – an excess of alkali

in the body (high pH number)

Remember, this chart shows foods that are acid

or alkali *forming* when digested. So, just because

the lemon might taste acidic, this does not mean

it is so after it has been combined with the

digestive juices. It does, in fact become alkaline –

hence its appearance, here, in blue.

PROTEINS AND FRUITS

Beef	Apples
Buttermilk	Apricots
Chicken	Avocados
Clams	Berries (all)
Cottage Cheese	Cantaloupes
Crab	Cranberries
Dairy Products	Currants
(except goat's milk)	Dates
Duck	Figs
Eggs	Grapes
Fish	Grapefruit
Goose	Honey (pure)
Jelly	Lemons
Lamb	Limes
Lobster	Oranges
Mutton	Peaches
Nuts	Pears
Oyster	Persimmons
Pork	Pineapple
Rabbit	Plums
Seeds (cooked)	Prunes
Sugar (raw)	Raisins
Tomatoes	Rhubarb
(processed)	Tomatoes (raw)
Turkey	
Turtle	
Veal	

NON-STARCH FOOD (VEGETABLES)

Alfalfa	Kelp
Artichokes	Kohlrabi
Asparagus	Leek
Aubergines	Lettuce
Beans (string)	Mushrooms
Beans (wax)	Okra
Beets (whole)	Olives (ripe)
Beet Leaves	Onions
Broccoli	Parsley
Cabbage (white)	Parsnips
Cabbage (red)	Peas (fresh)
Carrots	Peppers (sweet)
Carrot Tops	Radishes
Cauliflower	Rutabagas
Celery	Savory
Chicory	Seeds (sprouted)
Coconut	Sea Lettuce
Corn (raw)	Sorrel
Cucumbers	Soybean (products)
Dandelions	Spinach
Endives	Sprouts
Garlic	Summer Squash
Greens (leafy)	Swiss Chard
Horseradish	Turnips
Kale	Watercress

STARCHY FOODS

Bananas	Peas (Dried)
Barley	Potatoes (Sweet)
Beans (lima)	Potatoes (White)
Beans (white)	Pumpkin
Beans (kidney)	Quinoa
Breads (all)	Rice (Brown)
Buckwheat	Rice (White)
Cakes (all)	Rye Flour
Cereals	Sauerkraut
Chestnuts	Squash
Chick peas	Tapioca
Cookies (all)	Wheat Flour
Corn (processed)	(all, including Spelt,
Corn Meal	Semolina and
Corn Starch	Couscous)
Crackers	
Grapenuts	
Gluten Flour	
Lentils	
Macaroni (any)	
Millet Rye	
Oatmeal	
Pasta (any)	
Peanuts	
Peanut Butter	

FOODS TO AVOID

If you want your body to perform all the daily physical and emotional tasks that you require of it, you need to spend a little bit more time nurturing it and thinking about what you put into your system. And you need to know which are the food culprits and why you should avoid them. Know your enemy!

ARTIFICIAL FOODS

Refined foods often have toxic effects upon the body because of their acidic properties. Such foods include alcohol, fried and spicy foods, red meat, orange and grapefruit juice, tea, coffee, tomato ketchup, vinegar and mustard, to name but a few.

Fizzy drinks (anything that's carbonated) are valueless to the body and full of chemicals. They are what I call 'hollow foods' and are nutrition free. They also fill the digestive system with gas, causing bloating and acid in the blood.

Sugar, chocolates, cakes, biscuits, croissants are (I don't have to tell you) not allowed on Detox Programme – not just because of the their empty calories and their very low nutritional content, but also because they are crammed with fats, artificial sweeteners and refined sugars. Refined sugar is particularly bad because it has had all the goodness stripped away. The sweeteners create a yo-yo effect with our blood-sugar levels that impairs normal metabolism.

Baked beans, pizzas, spicy foods are also off the Detox list as they contain a lot of sugar or because they're loaded with saturated fats, or, in the case of deep fried and spicy foods because they're fatty and acidic.

Artificial flavourings (tomato ketchup, vinegar, sauces, pickles, mustards etc) are banned from the Detox Programme because of their acidic properties. They are dangerously full of hidden sugars, preservatives and artificial colouring – and many contain yeast.

Tea and coffee are also no-nos, not just because of their acidic properties but because of their artificial colourants and tannins which, when consumed in large quantities over long periods of time, can – among other things – make your teeth turn brown.

Tea and coffee also contain caffeine, the artificial stimulant which, as you will know, stimulates your metabolic rate. Caffeine is the reason you may have become addicted to coffee – particularly in the morning when you need jump-starting into action. The trouble is that caffeine makes your own natural stimulants (your thyroid and adrenal glands) redundant and lazy. Eventually, they cease to work properly and what was once a healthily stimulated metabolism becomes, instead, slow and sluggish.

FRUIT

Many fruits are only alkaline if picked when ripe. Because most of the fruit we buy in supermarkets is picked too early, it is highly acid-forming and lacking in nutrients. A recent BBC report about banana farmers in Ghana showed that, in order to comply with EC regulations, they had to use certain fertilizers and pesticide sprays that would allow the bananas to last at least two years! In addition to this, because I'm trying to encourage your body to get its energy from breaking down your fat stores (not from sugars, even if they are fruit sugars), and thereby releasing the toxins stored within them, I recommend forgoing fruit completely while on your three-week Detox.

The other reason I recommend avoiding fruit is because a lot of it is artificially sweetened, contains preservatives and is genetically modified, and so the only fruits that I advise are preferably organic and deliver a slow-release sugar boost – such as ripened bananas.

DEADLY NIGHTSHADES

You are also going to be avoiding foods belonging to the nightshade family – potatoes, aubergines, cucumbers, tomatoes and peppers – because of specific food intolerances that can occur over years. The nightshade family originates from the poison-ivy family and so is potentially poisonous to the body.

The members of this family are also acid-forming, even if they don't taste so. You may not think of potatoes as being acidic but, when you cut into a raw potato, watch how it slowly turns brown. That's the vitamin C, otherwise known as ascorbic acid, slowly oxidising. Cooking potatoes reduces their acidity – and that of tomatoes, which also have a high concentration of vitamin C.

Tomatoes pose a number of potential health problems. If, for instance, you are elderly and vulnerable to osteoporosis, having a high level of tomato in your system is going to mean that, to neutralise the acidity, your body will have to absorb calcium from your bones – which could bring on the bone-weakening condition of osteoporosis. Gout sufferers also have a high intolerance to tomatoes because the chemicals and nutrients they contain encourage a build up of the uric acid that causes the gouty pain. An excess of spicy foods, red meat, and red wine also has the same effect.

ALCOHOL

During the 21-Day Detox cut alcohol out completely. Once you are into the Maintenance Programme, if you are at a social function and it becomes difficult to resist a glass, then try opting for purer alcohols such as tequila, gin or vodka – but, remember, these are close relatives of your acid friends so beware of having too many! Another favourite alternative is a Cosmopolitan cocktail. To make one, you need: two measures of vodka, one measure of triple sec, one measure of lime juice, one measure of cranberry juice (unsweetened), ice and a strip of lime peel. Shake the ingredients together, pour into a Martini glass and garnish with lime.

Even though cranberries are quite acidic, they are very good for cystitis sufferers and have also been proved to be cardio-protective (due to their naturally occurring tannins which prevent thickening of the arteries). Don't imagine, though, that it's OK to drink vodka-based drinks as a nightly alternative to other alcohols. A Cosmopolitan is an emergency measure only!

YEAST, MOULDS AND FUNGI

One of the aims of the Detox Programme is to eliminate anything that has yeast or yeast preparations in it: soy sauce, pickles, Marmite, Vegemite, beer, bread, crackers, cereals etc. Yeasty foods tend to stick to your gut wall, sap energy and make you feel lethargic and bloated. Some people are also susceptible to developing the yeast disorder candidaisis, better known as candida, particularly if they eat a lot of yeast and are constipated. It sometimes affects those on the contraceptive pill because the candida (a yeast that lives in the intestine and other parts of the body) can grow and get out of control when hormonal balance is disrupted. Some of the more obvious symptoms of candida overgrowth are thrush, cystitis and fungal infections of the skin or nails.

I would suggest a close examination of your Ayurvedic Chart (in Chapter 6) to see whether you're a potential candida sufferer. If so, then stay away from any animal milk products, including goats' and sheep's milk, because they may contain certain bacteria that would exacerbate your condition; opt, instead, for rice milk and soya milk. If you are worried about your symptoms, then visit your GP.

It is also advisable to avoid mushrooms and certain nuts because they can encourage mould to harbour within the digestive system. Peanuts and pistachios are particularly problematic for this reason and are also high in calories and fatty oils. Walnuts and almonds are a good alternative.

If yeast, fungi, mould and bacteria are allowed to grow unchecked within the body, they will all claim first pickings of all the nutrients before the rest of your body gets a look in. Imagine that a waiter leaves a beautiful breakfast tray outside your holiday hotel room only for passing staff to start nibbling at your Danish and taking sips of your orange juice before you have even woken up! The yeast and mould inside your gut will behave just like the rogue hotel staff unless you see to it that they don't get a chance to linger.

DAIRY PRODUCTS

As far as possible, avoid dairy foods (cheese, milk, butter etc.) because they are both mucus-forming and acid-forming. (Full-fat cheese is also highly calorific.) Beware, too, of goats' milk and sheep's milk because they have similar properties. Opt instead for soya milk (unless you are menopausal) or rice milk.

RED MEAT

Red meat should be avoided because of its acidic properties. It also tends to be loaded with hormones and toxic matter that has either been fed to the animal or produced inside it as a chemical reaction. As soon as it becomes devoid of a normal blood supply, most red meat starts to decompose and rot, so it is important to understand that a piece of steak or a chop is something that has already started decaying. Red meat is difficult for the body to digest, particularly if it hasn't been chewed properly, which means valuable digestive energy is being spent on breaking it down rather than on nourishing our organs and blood supply. Red meat is also fattening and very high in cholesterol.

WHEAT AND GLUTEN

Other foods that you should also remove from your shelves for the 21-Day Detox period are bread, wheat and gluten products – including wheat pasta. Because of the gluey nature of the gluten, and the fact that it encourages a lot of mucus production within the gut, it hampers the digestion process and makes you feel sluggish. That doesn't mean to say that you can't have bread substitutes made from quinoa or spelt which don't contain much gluten.

I believe the reason why many people develop allergies to wheat and gluten is, in part, due to the way these grains are housed. Grain may be stored in warehouses for several years. During that time, mould can start to grow over the surface and, in time, will cover the entire granule. When the grain is eventually made into cereals or flour, a lot of the mould gets included in the process and it may very well produce allergic reactions.

Fortunately, most supermarkets now have sophisticated lines of gluten-free and wheat-free products. Try the gluten-free muesli without added sugar or fruit for breakfast with some rice (or perhaps soya) milk. But take care not to buy too many of these products; the muffins may be gluten-free and wheat-free, but they still contain calories.

MAKING POSITIVE FOOD CHOICES

It's not all about things to avoid though! I want you to feel energised and enthused by my Detox Programme, so take some inspiration from the abundance of foods available to you. Try experimenting and taking pleasure in preparing and eating your healthy meals – particularly during the working week, which may be your vulnerable time. Make a recipe plan from Monday to Friday – that way you won't be tempted to lunge for a bacon buttie or Kit Kat when those sugar cravings kick in. On a Monday, have a large salad with some smoked salmon. The next day, try grilled chicken with steamed vegetables. On Wednesday, make a vegetable soup and a stir-fry. On Thursday, boil some brown rice with some Tandoori chicken. And on Friday, prepare some sashimi – raw fish.

Salads and vegetables

Salads and steamed vegetables, obviously, are allowed in vast quantities; but, once you finish the 21-Day Detox Programme and move onto the Maintenance Programme, remember to check your Ayurvedic Profile. If you're someone with an increased Vata constitution, avoid eating too many raw vegetables because they produce a lot of gas and will create a metabolic imbalance.

Experiment with these foods to see which suit you. If salads make you feel bloated, try steamed vegetables. Listen to your body. You will know what it likes because you will start to feel the benefits of improved energy levels, better concentration and lower stress levels. If you have to have a dressing on your salad, choose extra-virgin olive oil. You could, perhaps, mix it with a little bit of lemon juice. Lemon juice, in small quantities, is as I've said, alkalising for the body but, in larger quantities, it can become acidic.

Dark-green leafy vegetables

You can eat a forest-full of dark-green vegetables including cabbage, greens, spinach, broccoli and kale. Avoid avocados if you have high cholesterol, because they are quite high in cholesterol, too; taken in small quantities, however, they are fine. Remember, balance is the key. Just because you're doing this Detox Programme for three weeks doesn't mean you should have an avocado every day. Vary your palate and your plate.

EGGS

Eggs are allowed, although preferably no more than three or four a week. Eat them any way you like, but try not to add milk or butter. Try boiling, poaching, scrambling with soya milk or rice milk, or frying in a spit of virgin olive oil. (You'll find Recipes at the back of the book.)

VEGETABLE JUICES

Freshly prepared vegetable juices are a definite 'yes', but please be very careful that no fruit juices are added. Mixing fruit and vegetables together may lead to fermentation of the sugars in the fruit which will produce more gas in your gut. Keep them apart so that they can be digested separately.

SOYA AND TOFU

Experiment with tofu; it is not as dull as people make out. You can marinate it, stir-fry it, grill it and have it with a black bean sauce and some rice noodles. For vegans, it's a useful alternative to scrambled eggs. Try mixing tofu with bananas and a little soya milk: that makes a delicious smoothie.

CHEESE ALTERNATIVE

Buffalo mozzarella is a nice alternative to cheese if you're a cheese-aholic. Have that with an avocado with a drizzle of extra-virgin olive oil as a starter or for lunch. It's going to have a potentially less intolerant effect than would normal cheese. Alternatively, have a Greek salad with feta or ricotta, or some cottage cheese. If you are vegetarian and you need to maintain your levels of protein, these types of cheese are all very good because they're less acidic and also not fermented.

CEREALS, PULSES AND LENTILS

Pulses and lentils help to nourish the adrenals and kidneys, while chickpeas and mung beans are excellent liver cleansers. It's worth making the effort to include them – and dahls– in your daily diet. They are all high in protein which is necessary for good liver function and for the production of digestive enzymes. They are alkaline-forming and contain no fat. You can soak them overnight, boil them, and mix with leafy vegetables and salads.

You can make a delicious starter by boiling a portion of green lentils and mung beans for 15–20 minutes, then covering them and adding a pinch of salt and some coriander. Or just throw the lot into a salad. (See the Recipe section for more ideas.)

FISH

Fish is an important source of protein –and of phosphorous and potassium which are essential nutrients for the brain. However, it is also quite acidic. Oily fish, rich in essential fatty acids, is very good for producing healthy hormones and regulating blood-sugar levels.

Explore the wide variety of fish available rather than sticking to the one or two you know. Treat yourself to some carp, or halibut, or cod or wild salmon. Try to avoid small shellfish, prawns, mussels and oysters because they 'hoover' up all the rubbish on the ocean floor and are usually quite high in heavy metals. It's worth looking for places where they are organically farmed and cultured, in a controlled environment that's far from the petroleum waste disgorged by ships.

I advise avoiding large marine fish, such as tuna and swordfish, because they do tend to absorb a lot of heavy metals; indeed, tuna is known to contain fairly toxic levels of mercury and lead.

BROWN RICE

I recommend replacing white rice, in your diet, with brown because it is rich in fibre and is far less glutinous. It is the least allergenic of all the varieties and is excellent for the nervous and digestive systems. It also has an exfoliating effect on the gut wall.

SOUPS

Vegetable soups are best home made from fresh organic vegetables, so avoid ones offered in even the smartest supermarkets because even the best will contain sugar and additives. Instead, take a pan of water, add some Brussels sprouts, peas, broccoli, asparagus and spinach. Keep stirring until it boils and then blend it into a wonderful vegetable consommé. Add a dash of pepper – and there you go. You can make a big batch and freeze it to last you the week. Wholesome soups make delicious meals, hot or cold; they are easy for the body to digest and full of rich, easily-absorbed nutrients.

DETOXIFYING SPICES

Black pepper: very aromatic when freshly ground. Gives food a 'bite'. It is effective in warding off colds and throat infections.

Cardamom/Cinnamon/Nutmeg: mostly ground down into a fine powder and used almost always in desserts containing milk. Cardamom prevents the formation of kidney stones, cinnamon is said to help fight diabetes and food poisoning, and nutmeg helps relieve stress.

Cloves: used whole in rice or meat dishes, and sometimes in baked foods. It controls gum and tooth infections, is anti-nausea, combats colds, strengthens nerves and improves the circulation.

Coriander: the most widely used garnish because it enhances the freshness and flavour of any dish. It cures indigestion and the seeds can reduce cholesterol.

Cumin: one of the main seasoning ingredients in curries. It is a good digestive and especially good at settling the stomach after a heavy meal.

Garlic: has a distinct sharp taste and aroma. A great complement to ginger and both are widely used together in Indian cuisine. It lowers cholesterol, inhibits rheumatism, and has anti-cancer, anti-flatulent and anti-bacterial/parasitic properties.

Ginger: has a distinct sharp taste and aroma. It improves digestion, lowers cholesterol, controls blood pressure, inhibits cancer, prevents coughs and colds, and has anti-nausea and anti-clotting properties.

Red chilli: gives curries and gravies their irresistible looks and 'hot' flavour. It is useful in that it stops you eating too much. It will however encourage the stomach to produce more acid.

Saffron: the most expensive spice in the world. It gives a beautiful glow to cuisine generally and an exclusive flavour to rice, meats, seafood and desserts. It is said to cure anaemia, it is an excellent nerve and heart tonic, and it has anti-aging properties.

Turmeric: used in Indian dishes. Imparts a rich look to the cuisine. It is a blood purifier, improves liver function, prevents coughs/colds, improves skin tone and is an antiseptic.

OLIVE OIL

Olive oil is a detox staple for re-establishing the correct ratio between the good and bad fats in your body. Good fats are essential for producing hormones and enzymes. They are called 'unsaturated fats' and are found in foods such as sunflower and pumpkin seeds, fish, vegetables, nuts and grains. Bad fats are saturated and found in red meat, margarine and dairy produce. Consumed frequently, saturated fats will increase your cholesterol levels, increase your weight and clog up your arteries. All of this can lead to heart disease.

Olive oil – or any cold-pressed oil such as sunflower, flaxseed or sesame – is rich in fatty acids, which are essential for good health, hormone balance and a well-nurtured complexion.

SALT AND SPICES

I do allow salt and pepper in moderation. Too much salt can increase blood pressure and debilitate the adrenal glands and kidneys. Many processed foods are high in salt and thus should be avoided. Certain spices, including turmeric, coriander and cumin, can be beneficial – not just for the flavour but because they're a natural digestive. You will find these spices widely used in Indian cookery, but not every spice is added to every single vegetable or meat dish. Each spice is selectively chosen for its flavour and properties. For example, turmeric is added in small quantities to a lot of vegetable and meat dishes because it aids digestion by encouraging the stomach's production of digestive gastric juices.

GOOD HABITS TO GET INTO

As well as avoiding certain foods and making positive choices about others, there are some really good basic habits you can adopt which will massively improve the effectiveness of the Detox Programme.

DRINKING WITH YOUR MEALS

All you need with meals is a glass of room-temperature water which will, as you sip it, allow a small amount of moisture to be mixed with the food. The watery medium enables the enzymes to work more effectively in breaking down the food's nutrients. This, in turn, allows the nutrients to be more easily digested and absorbed. It is much harder for the body to absorb and digest dried food – in just the same way as a canvas cannot absorb dry paint. Un-moistened food is also more likely to stick to the gut and colon. On the other hand, too much fluid can dilute your digestive enzymes and make them less able to do their job.

ALKALINE BREATHING

A little-known fact is that long, slow breathing makes us alkaline while rapid breathing makes us acid. The concentration of acid in our system can undermine our health. This acidity is a function of how many hydrogen ions (H+) we have in our tissue fluids and blood, and the concentration of these ions is directly related to our breathing oxygen.

TAKING IT SLOW

Take time over your meals – and think about what you are eating. If you can get away from your desk, or from slouching in front of the television, then sit at a table. Enjoy the flavour of each mouthful and resolve to chew each morsel enough times (at least eight to twelve) for the nutrients to be released and sent on a smooth passage to the stomach where they can be digested.

Try, also, to have smaller but more frequent meals to make sure that your body is continuously digesting food (which burns calories) and also to ensure that you maintain a healthy blood sugar level throughout the day. This will stop you experiencing sugar cravings and keep your energy levels up. Furthermore, it will also encourage your body to burn fat rather than muscle when you exercise, which will help you lose those inches off your waist and hips.

CHAPTER 4
DETOX LIQUIDS

A GOOD NUTRITIONAL PROFILE REQUIRES US TO EAT THE RIGHT KIND OF FOODS: CLEAN AND PURE AND FREE FROM ADDITIVES, PRESERVATIVES AND MAN-MADE CHEMICALS. IT ALSO DEMANDS AN INTAKE OF LIQUIDS THAT ARE EQUALLY CLEAN AND PRESERVATIVE FREE.

WE ARE COMPOSED OF 70–80 PER CENT WATER WHICH IS NOT ONLY NEEDED FOR SUSTAINING THE SHAPE OF OUR ORGANS, THE VOLUME OF OUR BLOOD AND THE MEDIUM IN WHICH OUR DIGESTIVE PROCESS CAN TAKE PLACE, BUT IS ALSO VITALLY IMPORTANT FOR MAKING POSSIBLE THE CHEMICAL PROCESSES THAT ARE OCCURRING, IN THE BODY, MILLIONS OF TIMES EVERY SECOND. WE ALSO NEED WATER TO ABSORB, DILUTE AND EVENTUALLY ELIMINATE THE WASTE PRODUCTS FROM OUR BODIES.

ON THE WHOLE, PEOPLE JUST DON'T DRINK ENOUGH OF IT. AS A RESULT, THE WATER CONTAINED WITHIN THEIR NORMAL INTERNAL ENVIRONMENT WILL BECOME MORE AND MORE CONCENTRATED WITH TOXINS. WE ALL NEED TO REALISE THAT THERE IS NO REPLACEMENT FOR REGULARLY CONSUMING FRESH, CLEAN WATER THAT THE BODY CAN PROCESS EASILY AND THEN USE FOR FLUSHING OUT THOSE TOXINS.

WATER – EAU DE VIE

Water is, quite simply, essential to life. It is the most vital constituent in our body – there would be no you or me without the existence of an ample water supply on Earth. The water content of the brain is 70 per cent, blood is made up of 82 per cent, and the lungs contain nearly 90 per cent.

The scope of water's uses is immense. It regulates temperature, removes toxins and waste products, assists in the digestion and absorption of food and allows for transportation of oxygen and nutrients to every cell. Every enzymatic and chemical reaction that takes place within your body occurs in the presence of water. It is also nature's best moisturiser; it hydrates the skin, as opposed to chemical face creams that simply seal in the moisture that is already there.

Water, which has a neutral pH value of 7, is called the 'universal solvent' because it dissolves more substances than any other liquid. This means that wherever water goes, either through the ground or through our bodies, it takes valuable chemicals, minerals, and nutrients along with it. But it's not just the minerals in the water that you need, it's the water itself.

DETOXING NECESSITY

You are capable of making some water in your own body, but not enough to match the losses incurred in urine, sweat and respiration. To remain in good health, you need to be drinking at least two litres a day. This will cleanse and purify you of all the chemicals and toxins that you continually ingest, absorb and inhale from our environment. Maintaining this water content will allow your kidneys to filter far better, help to prevent constipation and, if you're a woman, keep you free of cystitis infections.

It is also one of the most important weapons in the dieters' armoury. Cold water speeds up the body's metabolic rate due to the body's need to re-heat itself afterwards. So, the more water you drink, the greater the amount of calories your body burns up.

It is important that the daily quota is not made up of fruit juices or fizzy drinks as your body then has to extract the water out of the fluid before it can clean the system. In all likelihood, that water will then be needed to neutralise the effects of the sugars and preservatives contained within these type of drinks. Meanwhile, the water in drinks containing caffeine, which is a diuretic, such as tea or coffee, or in alcohol, will send you to the loo and so have the opposite effect of dehydrating, rather than hydrating, you.

DEHYDRATION

If your body becomes used to receiving insufficient fluid, it will learn to conserve what it's got and make do with the little it's getting. As a result, you may not be feeling thirsty when you could actually benefit enormously from drinking a great deal more.

The easiest way to monitor your current state of hydration is to check your urine. If it is pale, then there is enough water in your system. If it is deep yellow or orange, then you need to increase your water intake.

There is evidence that long-term mild dehydration is associated with various adverse health consequences. It is, therefore, important to keep to the optimum fluid intake. During hot weather or exercise it is important to replace water losses as much as possible by drinking at every opportunity.

EXERCISE, WATER AND GLYCOGEN

Heavy exercise also depletes muscle glycogen. This glycogen is the form of glucose, or simple sugar, that is stored in the liver and muscle and then used for generating energy. Every gram of glycogen holds about 2.5 to 3 grams of water so, when exercising, it is advisable to supply the body with extra glucose to help stimulate water absorption. There are a number of sports energy drinks that contain artificial sugars, but it is best, wherever possible, to get your glucose supply from natural sources such as fruit and vegetables. Ideally, instead of one of these drinks take carrot juice with you when exercising. If you don't want to make your own, there are a number of brands now readily available in high-street stores. Always opt for ones free of chemicals and preservatives.

DIFFERENT TYPES OF WATER

It is not just the amount of water that is important, but also the type. There's a whole range of different waters on the market nowadays: sparkling, still, mineral, spring and flavoured. Beyond that, you have the choice of plain, humble, tap water or water that's been filtered. They all have different properties, but which is best?

Mineral and spring water

You can get water, virtually free, from your kitchen tap, so what is the point of spending good money to get a bottle of mineral water? Well, many of us decide to do so because we believe that bottled water is a more natural and pure, alternative – even though blind taste tests have constantly proved that people cannot tell the difference between bottled and tap.

Both tap and bottled waters are 'ground waters' in that they started out as rain that seeped through rocks before collecting in underground pools. For water to be classed as 'mineral' it must come from a naturally protected source recognised by the local authority. It has a unique mineral content, depending on the geological area it has been drawn from, which must remain constant and be printed on the bottle.

Mineral water must be naturally free of dangerous bacteria and pollution. However, because it cannot be treated in any way that might alter its chemical composition, there is no way of gauging whether it has been contaminated by chemicals in the atmosphere or lead nitrates from fertilisers.

Spring water also comes from an underground source but it can be treated to remove impurities and pollutants and does not have to specify its mineral content on the bottle.

Storage of bottled water

Bottled water can spend up to two years sitting on shelves, in artificial packaging, before finally being drunk. Over time, as it sits in stuffy warehouses and warm supermarkets, the water will inevitably absorb some of the properties of that packaging. Also, there is a significant chance of microbes beginning to form within the liquid. Consumer tests that have been carried out on different types of bottled water have, in fact, shown that some bottled waters contain a greater accumulation of microbes than a glass of tap water.

There are no legal limits for bacteria in bottled waters, although there is a legal requirement that no bacteria must be introduced during the bottling process. The bacterium usually present is *Pseudomonas fluorescens*, found widely in fresh-water springs and not classed as a contaminant.

The major difficulty with bottled water is that we just don't know what is in it. Tap-water regulations make it mandatory that the public water supply is tested daily and that findings are freely available for scrutiny. There are no similar regulations for mineral and spring waters. What we do know, however, is that bottled mineral and spring waters have no health-giving properties over tap water. We also know that, while most bottled waters are safe, their mineral, chemical and bacterial content means that they are not *as* safe as tap water – yet, they cost around 1,500 times as much. I recommend drinking tap water over bottled water but ensure you have a good filter system, either integrated with your tap or as a separate stand-alone jug, and make sure you change the filter as regularly as necessary. There is, therefore, an anomalous situation where different regulations apply to what is essentially the same commodity, water, which is merely packaged in a different way. Bottled waters should be subject at least to the same regulations as tap

water. It could be argued, however, that if their advertising is going to stress their inherent purity, and if they are to cost so much more, perhaps their regulations should be even more stringent. There is little doubt that if tap-water regulations were applied to bottled waters, many would disappear from supermarket shelves. Furthermore, the chemicals contained in the plastic of plastic bottles have been linked to infertility in women; so, if you prefer mineral or spring water to tap, I recommend that you buy it in a glass bottle wherever possible.

Sparkling versus still

Sparkling water appears to be seen, by some people, as a fashion accessory. I don't recommend it because, even if it's naturally carbonated, that carbon will render the water slightly acidic. It can even work against the detoxification process. Taking carbonated water into your system is going to increase gas formation that can lead to bloating and other digestive disorders, and the acidic content might irritate your stomach lining. I would, therefore, always opt for still water, of any type, over sparkling.

Fruit waters

Waters flavoured with mango, apple, peach, blackcurrant, and numerous other fruit and combinations thereof, are increasingly popular. Again, these are not products I would recommend because the fruit flavouring that is added to the water is a synthesized chemical. Patients come to me with headaches or joint aches, believing they have been making a healthy choice in drinking these flavoured waters without realising that the artificial chemicals in them are causing their symptoms. It is also going to cause the liver unnecessary stress since it has to extract the water it needs from these chemical additives (which include sugars).

MINERAL WATER CONTENTS

Here's a quick rundown of all the minerals found in mineral waters and exactly why you need them:

Bicarbonate: regulates the body's acidity.

Calcium: good for bones and also for muscle activity.

Fluoride: needed for healthy teeth and helps protect the cardiovascular system.

Iron: essential to make red blood cells, which take oxygen around the body.

Magnesium: for some people, magnesium is very helpful for menstrual cramps. It is also especially good for people with heart problems as it relaxes the muscles of the vascular system.

Potassium: helps control blood pressure. Although having too much salt is blamed for high blood pressure, the body's having insufficient potassium can also be the cause.

Silica: needed for strong bones, fingernails and hair.

Sodium chloride: helps maintain a normal fluid volume in the body. Required for digestion, muscular function and the nervous system.

Sulphate: assists in producing haemoglobin – the vital constituent of red blood cells that facilitates the blood's uptake of oxygen.

Zinc: boosts the immune system.

Tap water

Tap water is a cocktail of water made up from recycled domestic waste, rainwater and surface water from rivers, lochs, and reservoirs. The initial untreated water contains dirt, waste, pieces of leaves and other organic matter, as well as trace amounts of certain contaminants. Chemical coagulants are added to the water as it flows, very slowly, through the treatment tanks, so that all the particles and impurities form clumps that settle on the bottom. The water is then passed through a filter for removal of even the smallest contaminants such as viruses and giardia (a parasite that can cause stomach upsets). This filtering process is repeated several times because water in the UK has to be cleaned to a very high standard.

Before 1980, there were few regulations for tap water. Recent advances in equipment sophistication have meant that previously unknown substances are now being detected in tap water. Nevertheless, the high standard of water production in the UK does not mean that we shouldn't exercise caution.

It is not the products that are taken out of tap water that worry me so much as the chemicals that are then added to it, including chlorine, aluminium, and fluoride. What particularly alarms me, however, are prescription drugs. Urine is one of the ways that the body rids itself of toxins, but a huge number of us are expelling vast quantities of these chemicals that are then recycled back into our drinking water. Women, particularly, are passing large amounts of hormones such as progesterone through taking the contraceptive pill, while both sexes are passing all sorts of anti-depressants and painkillers.

These chemicals may not actually be removed from the water during the filtering process and, over a period of months or even years they can build up to a concentration that could have implications for the health of the body. That puts further stress on the liver and the kidneys and affects our hormonal status and general wellbeing. So, while tap water is absolutely fine for washing salads and vegetables, I wouldn't advise drinking it regularly in large quantities unfiltered.

Hard versus soft

Hard water is the normal water that tends to flow from our taps. Soft water has had salt added to it. When you add salt to the water, calcium bicarbonate is formed. This softens the water and it becomes more beneficial for bathing. People with soft water find they use less cleaning solutions when washing clothes or dishes and, because the salt neutralises the calcium in the water, it prevents appliances from developing scale and lime deposits. However, soft water is not suitable for drinking.

Filtered tap water

Because of the overwhelming number of different chemicals and contaminants that can be found in today's water supply – and the problems with bottled water already mentioned – my first choice is filtered tap water because it is the purest.

You can buy various filters that reduce chlorine, ammonia, and lime-scaling calcium deposits, help rid the water of microbes, and even change the pH value so as to make it more acidic or alkaline.

The most advanced of these is a reverse-osmosis filter that uses a technique perfected by the space station, NASA, to purify fluids on lunar modules, and which removes all salts, chemicals and minerals. The result is a completely pollution-free liquid, but even using the most basic filters will be an improvement on drinking water straight out of the tap.

One simple example which shows the levels of toxins in our drinking water is the presence of lime scale. If you make a herbal tea with tap water, you will probably find that, as the tea settles, the liquid develops a film on the top. This is calcium lime scale, a substance that will then be deposited within your kidney tubules where it can potentially cause blockages, and also in your blood vessels which can encourage hardening of the arteries.

Filters help to reduce all of this rubbish and bacteria, but it is important to keep filtered water in a cool place or microbes will start growing in it. The same caution applies to bottled water. To illustrate the point, if you were to leave some water sitting around, after five to ten days it will become slimy with tiny organisms floating in it. Obviously, you wouldn't drink the water after this amount of time, but even after a few days these microbes will have started to develop and, if drunk, will decompose inside you, releasing their poisons in the process.

I cannot, therefore, overestimate the importance of the quality of the water that you drink. Most of us assume that drinking the correct amount is enough. In fact, drinking the right type of water can make an enormous difference to your sense of wellbeing which is why I would always suggest that, if possible, you drink filtered.

FIONA'S STORY

Even though I have dieted all my life, over the years I have gradually piled on the weight to the point that I was 13st 2lb – and I am only 5ft 2in. I didn't want to go out and buy clothes because I was so overweight. I always wanted to wait until the next diet and that time when I was going to lose all that weight but, of course, it just never happened. And it wasn't just the weight that was bothering me, it was the fact that I had no energy. The only thing that was keeping me going was my brain. I had to drag myself around by pure will power.

I began the diet with an open mind and I was also very positive. I stuck to it rigidly. Two days after I started, I was sick. I think it was just toxic overload. I also had a lot of headaches and, for the first few days, I just wanted to put my head down on my desk and sleep.

But then, very quickly, quite miraculous things started happening. First, I noticed that I was sleeping better. Then, I started wanting to get up in the morning. That had never happened before. Then I found myself running for the bus – and, in three weeks, I lost a stone.

I must admit that, in those three weeks, I did cheat a little bit. I had a bit of a wine and champagne binge at a social event – but I still lost weight and I wasn't hungry once. Nor was I craving anything; and now, I don't get the same cravings for carbs that I used to.

I didn't find the programme restrictive at all. Even during the stringent 21-day period, I went out to lunch and dinner quite often. It's quite easy to find things you can eat in a restaurant; there's always something in the way of a fish or chicken dish.

After about a week, people started commenting – not so much on the weight loss, but about how well I looked. They said my skin was glowing and that my eyes were sparkling. Of course, you swell up with pride and then you start to feel encouraged. Then people started noticing the weight.

I'm still following the Programme. I don't think of it as a diet at all. Well, it's not; it's now a way of life. I don't feel at all deprived. I was worried about missing coffee; I used to have three or four cups every day, and a morning cappuccino, but that was OK. And it's fine to have the odd treat although, to be honest, I don't enjoy them the way I once did. I always used to have an almond croissant and, after a few weeks, I was really looking forward to having one again; but it just didn't taste quite as good.

I hated my body before. I didn't like looking in a mirror. I don't hate it now. The other day, I bought a size 12 dress which made me feel great. As the weight starts going down so your confidence starts going up. The other thing I have noticed is that the Programme has had a pronounced effect on my physical environment. I've been clearing out my house, and my cupboards, because I got a strong feeling that I wanted to unload my material belongings, too.

FIONA SPENCER THOMAS IS A FREELANCE MARKETING EXECUTIVE IN HER LATE FORTIES. SHE LIVES IN LONDON AND IS MARRIED WITH A TEENAGE DAUGHTER.

FIZZY DRINKS

Carbonated mineral waters were first produced towards the end of the 18th century and flavoured versions, which eventually became soft drinks, were introduced during the 19th century. This is when phosphoric acid was added and colas were created.

Although they are fast, easy, and often thirst-quenching, there is absolutely nothing in fizzy drinks that provides us with any real nutritional value. The only natural ingredient in Coca Cola is water. Everything else in there is chemically produced, including the sugar. Years ago I carried out an experiment to monitor the effects of Coca Cola. I placed a chicken bone in a bowl of the drink and, after a week, it had completely dissolved. It isn't difficult to make the link to the human body and realise how potentially harmful these soft drinks can be. All the chemicals, artificial flavourings, additives and preservatives contained within them have to be processed by your liver which, as it becomes more and more congested, has to store the toxins it can't handle in your fat cells and within the liver cells themselves.

Women, especially, choose to drink low-calorie fizzy drinks because they help to curb the appetite on calorie-controlled diets. However, an article, published in *The Lancet* in 1991, revealed that cellulite is a very specialist form of fat cell that contains high levels of artificial sweeteners, so the price of suppressing your appetite is a build up of fat stores – and your cellulite levels.

The only fizzy drink that does have some sort of beneficial property is Indian tonic water because of the levels of quinine it contains. Quinine is a bitter-tasting drug obtained from the bark of the South American cinchona tree and has been used for centuries to prevent and treat malaria. It was added to tonic water because the drink was originally intended, in the colonial era, for consumption in the tropical areas of India and Africa where that disease was endemic.

Quinine does have an unusual number of benefits. It has been used medicinally to allay fever, to induce uterine contractions during labour, as a hardening agent in the treatment of varicose veins, and as a way of reducing cramps. If you find yourself suffering from cramp, then a 500ml glass of Indian tonic water, taken regularly, should be enough to relieve the muscle spasms.

COFFEE

In the UK, 80 per cent of adults drink coffee every week. As its name suggests, it has very high levels of caffeine although, interestingly, coffee beans actually contain half the amount of caffeine of tea leaves. A cup of coffee only has higher levels of caffeine than a cup of tea because it is drunk in a much more concentrated form.

Caffeine is a drug that acts as a stimulant to the heart and central nervous system, and is also known to increase blood pressure in the short-term. The stimulating effect of coffee peaks in the blood 15 to 45 minutes after drinking – but may persist for hours. How fast your body processes the caffeine depends on your metabolic rate and how sensitive you are, but its expulsion is slowed by pregnancy and medications including antacids and the Pill.

Caffeine is also a diuretic and can flush important chemicals, such as potassium, from the body as well as making you dehydrated. Meanwhile, heavy consumption of coffee boiled in a coffee-making machine has long been suspected of having a cholesterol-raising effect, although the evidence remains inconclusive.

All of these factors are damaging to our general wellbeing, but the main reason that I ban coffee on the Detox Programme is because it is very acidic and will upset the body's pH balance. I know that some people will find this very difficult. Caffeine, like nicotine (albeit to a lesser extent) meets some of the criteria of the World Health Organization and the American Psychiatric Association for a drug of dependence. It acts on the dopamine system in the same way as amphetamines and cocaine. Dopamine is a neurotransmitter – a brain chemical that carries messages between the brain cells. It is associated, in particular, with feelings of pleasure, usually after food or sex. Any drug, therefore, that artificially affects dopamine levels may cause a craving for more of that drug.

However, I'm afraid the only way to give up your daily cups of coffee is to wean yourself off them gently because decaffeinated varieties can be just as harmful. The decaffeination process has chemically altered their composition and, as a result, they will deposit unwanted toxins in the body that will put undue stress on the liver.

TEA

As a British Nutrition Foundation report of 1992 noted: "Until the 17th century, few non-alcoholic drinks were available and people mostly consumed ale, cider and wine. Herbal teas or infusions were consumed as medicines. By the 18th century, tea had became the most popular drink in the UK as it still remains today – we drink an estimated 196,000,000 cups every day – and it is the most commonly consumed beverage in the world after water."

There are three different types of tea: black, green and red (or oolong). They are all from the same plant, *Camelia sinensis*, but just processed in different ways. Black and red teas are partially dried, crushed and fermented, while green teas are briefly steamed.

The good old-fashioned cup of 'char' has more medical value than is usually assumed. It has shown some real benefits such as reducing heart disease and diminishing the risk of pancreatic, prostate, stomach and lung cancer. This is thanks to its range of vitamins, minerals and antioxidants that provide a good nutrition balance and also have anti-aging properties.

However, tea also contains caffeine so – as with coffee – it is a stimulant for the your heart and central nervous system, and can cause your blood pressure to rise (albeit short term). It also has a mild diuretic effect so I do not recommend black or red tea on the Detox programme.

HEALING GREEN TEA

I do, though, advise that you drink green tea, which is far less processed and has less caffeine. It also has a very high concentration of antioxidants including flavonoids and polyphenols which have numerous health-giving properties. Polyphenols, in particular, have been found to be 20 times more effective than the other antioxidant powerhouses, vitamins C and E.

The effects of these antioxidants are truly wide-ranging. When the starch of carbohydrates is consumed, it requires the enzyme amylase to break it down into simple sugars that can be absorbed into the bloodstream. Green tea polyphenols inhibit amylase and so can help lower blood-sugar levels and prevent diabetes. A recent study has also found that the green-tea antioxidants may prevent or reduce the severity of symptoms of rheumatoid arthritis because they inhibit the Cox-2 gene that triggers inflammation, working in much the same way as anti-inflammatory drugs.

The tea's antioxidants help the liver to function more efficiently. And because they help to control blood-sugar levels, they also lower the levels of the body's fat stores. (High blood-sugar levels are responsible for the storage of glucose as fat.)

Green tea can also help to lower blood pressure. A major cause of hypertension (high blood pressure) is an enzyme secreted by the kidneys called angiotension-converting-enzyme (ACE). Popular drugs for hypertension act as ACE inhibitors: by blocking the effects of ACE, blood pressure is reduced. Green tea is a natural ACE inhibitor, and several medical studies record lowered blood pressure in animals and humans when given green tea extracts.

Laboratory studies show that the polyphenols in green tea can help prevent some cancers and may stabilise or shrink present cancers, keeping them from spreading. This effect seems to lie in their ability to prevent the oxidation that damages DNA, turning normal cells into cancer cells. Most studies are laboratory based, and results in humans are inconclusive, but observational evidence is beginning to prove a link.

The only slight downside is that green tea does contains some caffeine so resist drinking it from late afternoon onwards – and certainly not just before bedtime. Opt for a variety of peppermint or camomile, instead. Camomile, lime blossom and lemon balm all encourage sleep, while peppermint, fennel, liquorice and ginger aid digestion. Ginseng tea will also energise and build stamina.

ALCOHOL

A lot of confusion surrounds the potential health benefits and dangers of alcohol consumption. There are some studies which suggest a glass of wine each day is good for thinning the blood, and researchers from Imperial College, London, have reported in the *British Medical Journal* that resveratrol, a component of red wine, has anti-inflammatory and antioxidant properties that can help treat a common type of lung disease.

For the purposes of the 21-Day Detox, I do not allow any alcohol. However, once you get on to the Maintenance Programme, although white wine, red wine, champagne, beer and lager are still off- limits, as all of these drinks are extremely acidic and high in yeast, you can allow small quantities of distilled alcohol such as gin and vodka. These purer alcohols are less harmful to the body and they also have fewer cogeners, the chemical by-products of fermentation that can produce headaches and dizziness. But, as with all alcoholic drinks, distilled alcohols can also inflict harm in the long term.

When swallowed, alcohol passes from the stomach to the digestive tract where it enters the bloodstream within minutes of consumption. Within an hour, 90 per cent of an alcoholic drink has been absorbed. It travels to every part of the body, especially the brain, liver and kidneys.

The opposite of caffeine, alcohol is a central nervous system depressant. It acts as a tranquilliser and mild anaesthetic, a use to which it's been put for centuries. No one knows exactly how alcohol exerts its effects, but it's thought to cause the release of naturally occurring pain relievers in the body (called opioids), that make people feel less inhibited and more relaxed.

However, in larger amounts, alcohol slows mental functions and can cause loss of memory, poor judgment, dizziness, poor co-ordination, slurring of speech, blurred vision, vomiting and, eventually, unconsciousness. It is, therefore, not surprising that, if abused, alcohol can cause a whole host of long-term problems including heart-disease, pancreatitis, nervous-system disorders, cancer and liver damage.

PHILIP'S STORY

I was introduced to Joshi by an Indian dancer friend. I visited him in his role as an osteopath because I had a neck injury which he cured after just two treatments. I went to see him again after I had a car accident that left me suffering from whiplash and, again, he sorted me out, but this time by using acupuncture. I have always been very cynical about alternative treatments but the acupuncture worked.

Then, I went to see him again, complaining of lots of aches and pains. I felt I was facing an early mid-life crisis. When I asked him what he thought my problem was he said, "You are getting fat. You need to lose about ten kilos". I weighed about 14½ stone and was 5ft 11in. I was chunky but never thought I was fat, so I was quite taken aback. I had tried various diets before but, of course, none of them worked and they only gave me headaches.

He recommended his Detox programme and I followed it to the letter for six weeks – 21 days on the Detox and 21 on the Maintenance Programmes. It worked extremely well for me. I even took up running which I had never done before. Joshi said that exercise was a vital part of the Detox. I lost a stone in six weeks. People said I looked better. I felt very good, too. The key benefit was that I was able to work and think faster and more effectively.

I was impressed because Joshi looked after me holistically which is why I found it easier to keep on with the Detox. It gave me something to hang on to as it was changing my life – I started running every morning, composing music more fluently, managing my life more effectively, and sleeping better but needing less. I was amazed I managed to come off coffee, alcohol and sweet things without it finishing me off. I was addicted to caffeine and I like wine but I didn't really miss them.

The new way of eating also lowered my appetite massively in that I wouldn't want a second plate of food. I would eat smaller portions of food more frequently. I do work long hours, sometimes 12-hour days non-stop from 8am to 8pm so I graze on rice cakes and biscuits that are gluten free and wheat free – things that take more energy to eat than give you energy, perhaps. Joshi also detoxed my head, which was fantastic; I can't believe how it cleared my brain. Now, I feel great all over. My wife is amazed too. I didn't used to feel in control of my life in that I had to juggle so many things, but now I have the energy to keep everything in balance and in control. I have been able to write a book, compose a symphony, teach students, practice and play in concerts – and still have time for my family and friends. Joshi's Detox gave me the kick my body needed. I will never go back to eating the way I did. Now I don't even like desserts, and no more than a glass and a half of wine is fine for me. The last time I felt this well was when I was 19 and living off rice, raw fish and green tea in Japan.

PHILIP SHEPPARD, 35, IS A CELLO PROFESSOR AT THE ROYAL ACADEMY OF MUSIC AND IS NOW TRAINING FOR THE LONDON MARATHON. HE IS MARRIED WITH TWO YOUNG DAUGHTERS AND LIVES IN BUCKINGHAMSHIRE.

MILK AND DAIRY PRODUCE

For most of the last century, milk has been prized as a cornerstone of a healthy diet. And it's true that milk is an important, nutritionally dense food that provides us with an excellent source of protein, calcium, (essential for strong bones), vitamins such as riboflavin, vitamin A and vitamin D (necessary for cardiovascular health and energy production), and iodine (a mineral essential for thyroid function).

Milk is available in many forms: whole, raw, skimmed, semi-skimmed and UHT. Raw milk is milk that has not been pasteurised. The difference between whole milk, low-fat milk, and fat-free milk (and similar dairy products) is the fat and calorie content. Fat-free milk and milk products have the same amount of protein, vitamins and minerals (including calcium) as whole milk; what they don't have is the saturated fat and extra calories. UHT milk stands for Ultra High Temperature milk which is put through a heating process that kills 100 per cent of any form of bacterial growth so it can be packaged for up to nine months at a time.

Since the 1970s, our milk intake has steadily decreased and this has been blamed, in turn, for the equivalent decrease in our calcium levels – a decrease which means that one in three women now suffer from osteoporosis. However, according to recent research, the bone loss and deteriorating bone tissue that occur in osteoporosis are not due to calcium deficiency but to the fact that our bodies are excreting too much of the calcium they already have.

The reasons for this loss of calcium are thought to be the over-consumption of protein and a generally acidic diet. Foods such as meat, eggs – and dairy – make excessive demands on the kidneys as they try to eliminate their waste products (urea). During this process, calcium is leached from the body – the calcium that is needed for healthy teeth, bones and body tissue. In other words, rather than protecting against weak and brittle bones and diseases such as osteoporosis, milk could turn out to be their cause. Consuming too much milk can, therefore, actually be bad for you.

This might explain why American women are among the biggest consumers of calcium in the world but still have one of the highest levels of osteoporosis. The Chinese consume little or no dairy foods and get all their calcium from vegetables and fish. They consume only half the calcium of Americans yet osteoporosis is uncommon in China, despite an average life expectancy of 70 years.

Recent studies have shown that, except for people of northern-European origin, most adults the world over can't digest lactose, the natural sugar in milk. This needs to be broken down by the enzyme lactase that lives in our intestines and bowels. If we absorb more lactose than we can digest, the surplus travels to the large intestine where it ferments, producing gas, carbon dioxide and lactic acid. These symptoms will, in turn, cause indigestion, bloating, cramps, nausea, tiredness and diarrhoea. More and more people are developing lactose intolerance, as our bodies give up trying to make enough of the enzyme that breaks lactose down. This is why I favour such alternatives such as goats' milk, rice milk and soya milk.

If a person is lactose intolerant but would like to drink small amounts of milk, I would recommend skimmed or semi-skimmed as they have high nutrient levels with low levels of saturated fat. However, for the 21 days of the Detox Programme, I will be taking you off dairy completely because it is very mucus-forming and tends, therefore, to allow the body to harbour toxins within the digestive system.

GOATS' MILK

Goats' milk is a natural alternative to cows' milk and has 25 per cent more vitamin B-6, 47 per cent more vitamin A, 134 per cent more potassium and 350 per cent more of niacin (a B-complex vitamin). Goats' milk is also higher in certain essential fatty acids (linoleic and arachidonic acids) and in the essential minerals chloride, copper and manganese, and it contains 27 per cent more of the essential nutrient selenium.

Like cows' milk, goats' milk does contain lactose but it can be drunk by many people who suffer from cows'-milk allergies or sensitivity. Goats' milk casein curd (protein) is both softer and smaller than that produced by bovine milk, and so it is more easily accepted by the human digestive system. It also has smaller-sized fat globules that provide a better dispersion, and a more homogenous mixture, of fat in the milk – making it easier to digest.

Because goats' milk is more easily absorbed, it leaves less undigested residue behind in the colon. It is this residue that ends up fermenting in the system and causing the uncomfortable symptoms of lactose intolerance. However, if you still suffer a lot from bloating, cramps, or digestive disorders, it means that you are sensitive to goats' milk and would do well to avoid it.

SOYA MILK

Soya is the only vegetable that contains all the amino acids found in meat, fish, or eggs. If you are vegetarian, it's particularly important to include large quantities of it in your diet in order to get the full spectrum of amino acids. These are vital for hormone production and to boost the immune system. Soya milk does, however, lack some of the essential elements of cows' milk, so do select a brand fortified with calcium and vitamins A and D.

Soya has been hailed as a wonder solution for several conditions, including heart disease, breast and prostate cancer, menopausal symptoms and bone health. This is because it is rich in oestrogen-like substances known as isoflavones. They appear to help counter-balance the declining levels of oestrogen as we age, protecting against disease and preserving the youthful appearance of your skin. Isoflavones also have strong antioxidant properties, and soya is a source of soluble fibre that can lower cholesterol levels.

Recently, it has been found that soya can destabilise the female hormonal cycle, giving women hot flushes and possibly bringing their menopause forward. It seems that it doesn't just change the oestrogen in a woman's body but the progesterone levels as well, thus cancelling out any good side effects. While I do recommend soya milk as a good cows' milk substitute, particularly for vegetarians, it should be consumed in controlled amounts. If you are menopausal, pre-menopausal or have fluctuating periods, avoid soya milk because it could have an effect on your hormonal balance. The best alternative for you would be rice milk.

RICE MILK

Made from brown rice and filtered water, rice milk has a light, slightly sweet flavour that substitutes well for all other milks. It is 100 per cent lactose free and suitable for all those people who are sensitive to dairy products. However, rice milk is not a nutritional replacement for cows' milk. It is important that you choose a product that is fortified with essential iron and calcium and also make sure that you include alternative sources of protein in your diet.

YOGHURT

Yoghurt was one of the very first 'health' foods and is still one of the best. It is high in calcium needed to build healthy bones, it supplies the B vitamins, B12 and folic acid, which help to build a healthy blood supply and contains 'friendly' bacteria which can assist in keeping a healthy gut.

When I talk about yoghurt, I always mean plain live (or 'bio') yoghurt as that contains the *Bifidobacteria* and *Lactobacillus acidophilus* bacteria which naturally reside in the gut lining and are excellent aids to good digestion. The fruit-flavoured non-bio versions that you will often find in supermarkets are not nutritious foods. They are pumped with preservatives, chemicals, additives and artificial sugars, and are a complete no-no for a healthy balanced diet.

Yoghurt's probiotics

Yoghurt's bacteria or microbes are collectively known as probiotics, literally 'pro life' indicating that they help rather than harm. In particular, they inhibit the growth of *Helicobacter pylori*, a bacterium linked with peptic ulcers and stomach cancer.

Probiotics can also reduce overgrowth of candida in the gut – the yeast responsible for recurrent thrush infections – and improve symptoms of irritable bowel syndrome such as constipation, diarrhoea and bloating. A healthy gut that is teeming with good bacteria helps the body to absorb calcium, too, thus lessening the risk of developing osteoporosis. Live yoghurt is also an effective way of combating gas and bloating as the 'good' bacteria force out the bad gas-producing bacteria.

Yoghurt for soothing and cleansing

Having a bio yoghurt every morning will help the normal bacteria in your stomach to repopulate on a daily basis. In turn, this will help to clean the digestive system of microbes and any bacteria that you may ingest during the day.

One very good Ayurvedic or Indian remedy, for settling an upset stomach is to make a yoghurt drink. Take a couple of tablespoons of live yoghurt, mix with water, add a pinch of salt and a pinch of ground up cumin and drink.

Live yoghurt is also an excellent cleanser for people who are prone to acne and spots because it clears away any bacteria which might otherwise infect the sebaceous glands. You can use it as a face mask, as well as eating it.

If you wish to have a fruit yoghurt then add your own – although for the 21-Day Detox Programme, the only fruit I allow are bananas. Later, you can move onto a range of different fruits as long as they are not too acidic including apples, apricots, berries, grapes, peaches, pears and oranges. While these fruits are alkaline-forming when ripe, most of the time they are picked before they are ripe which is when they are acid-forming.

JUICES

Juicing is the quickest, most effective, way of providing the body with all the vitamins, minerals and enzymes that are essential for good health and increased vitality. You may be surprised to learn that it's not easy to achieve the recommended daily allowance of nutrients – not even if you eat fruit and take the time to prepare fresh meals with a good proportion of vegetables. Cooking for instance, although an invaluable tool that can increase the antioxidant activity of some vegetables, does reduce the levels of some enzymes and certain nutrients such as the water-soluble B and C vitamins.

WHY JUICE?

Juices use raw vegetables and they also enable you to absorb large quantities of nutrients at a time. Once you get into juicing, the likelihood is that you will buy and consume a great deal more fruit and vegetables than before. You probably wouldn't have considered eating 1lb of carrots a day but, within minutes, what would have previously seemed like a week's supply can be transformed into an 8oz glass of zesty juice that will have an almost miraculous effect on your well-being. Not only will that juice furnish you with increased energy and strengthened immunity, it will flush the toxins out of your body, provide the raw materials to help you heal more quickly and completely – and it is low calorie, practically fat-free and bursting with vitamins and minerals.

Fresh juices also provide essential enzymes and a concentrated source of the antioxidant vitamins A (converted by the body from beta carotene), C and E. Enzymes are the body's work force, acting as the catalyst for the hundreds of thousands of chemical reactions that take place every day – from the digestion and absorption of food to the production of energy – while the antioxidants mop up excess 'free radicals', the rogue molecules that attack cells and tissues and are linked with heart disease and cancer.

Because they are so fast acting, juices act a little bit like a blood transfusion. During the juicing process all the fibre is removed from the vegetable leaving the vitamin- and mineral-rich pulp that is then absorbed directly into the bloodstream. Within 20 minutes, this vital source of energy is nourishing the body's cells. It is good to juice the whole vegetable because the skin contains certain nutrients and bacteria that will help the body digest the juice.

By fresh juices, I do not mean those items labelled 'fresh' on supermarket shelves which are, in fact, watery processed liquids that have been packed in cardboard or plastic and are full of chemicals, colourings and preservatives. Most of these pre-made juices have also been heated up to 175 degrees Fahrenheit for 20 to 30 minutes to extend their shelf-life, which means that most of the all-important enzymes and nutrients have been destroyed in the process. These are no substitute for real juice made from the fresh produce that will provide a wholesome, health-giving, drink that tastes delicious.

HOW TO JUICE

The most important piece of equipment is a juicer. Unlike a liquidiser or blender, this grates the unpeeled vegetables into a strainer basket which then spins the pulp to extract the juice. The juice runs out of the machine topped with a gorgeous cappuccino-style froth.

If you are new to juicing, start out with an inexpensive juicer. Then, if you decide you like it and want to juice regularly, invest in a more expensive model which will last for longer and will extract a greater quantity of juice from the pulp.

It's important to begin slowly with juices, because your body will not be accustomed to digesting such a concentrated form of nutrients. It is also better to drink juice on an empty stomach because that way it will pass into your intestine more quickly for an immediate vitamin and mineral boost.

One thing that you must remember is that raw, unpreserved juice is highly perishable, so try to drink juice immediately after making it. Any contact with light, heat or air will start an oxidation process that will eventually break down many of its valuable nutrients. However, if you would like to take juice to work, it can be kept in a thermos flask, or chilled in a fridge, for up to 6 hours.

It has been claimed that you can overdose on certain vegetables or vitamins. It is true that too much vitamin A and beta carotene in the bloodstream will result in an orangey complexion so, unless you are after a curious overall tan effect, vary your vegetables to get a broad spectrum of all the different minerals, enzymes, vitamins, and antioxidants available.

WHAT TO JUICE

Almost all fruits and vegetables can be juiced, but for the purposes of the 21-Day Detox Programme and establishing the body's correct acid/alkaline levels, I recommend that you only juice vegetables. You may think that a fruit snack is better than chocolate but, at this point of the Detox what you are doing is attacking your sugar craving with another sugar-containing food that is also fairly high in calories.

I also advise against mixing fruit and vegetables together. Patients of mine who complain of bloating tell me, rather proudly, that they drink an apple and carrot juice every morning. However, fruit and vegetable juices mixed together will start to ferment in the gut and this is what causes bloating. Carrot juice is already quite sweet and so the apples are really not necessary for flavour. Instead, add some ginger which will give it a new kick and stimulate the liver function.

The easiest way to start juicing is with vegetables that you like to eat non-juiced. Once you have got a taste for single juices – carrot, beetroot, celery, for instance – you can start being a bit more creative. Mix together some beetroot and carrot. Add a squeeze of lemon or some fresh parsley. The key to juicing is to experiment with it. Other vegetables that make great juices are fennel, Jerusalem artichokes and parsnips, and also leafy greens such as spinach, parsley and sprouts.

Juice is the ultimate fast food. You can take a whole carrier bag of fresh organic produce and absorb all the nutritional content that it has to offer in just a few glasses of juice. However – although this may be tempting – you must not eat all your fruit and vegetables in this way. Juices do not contain fibre so they should never completely replace whole fruits and vegetables in your diet.

WHEATGRASS – THE SPECIAL INGREDIENT

Wheatgrass is well known in holistic healing circles for its therapeutic effect in fighting cancer, on blood purification, liver detoxification and colon cleansing. Drinking wheatgrass juice will provide the body with a superb source of chlorophyll – the unique element in plants that traps sunlight energy and which has, therefore, a vast range of vitamins and minerals.

However, because it is such a potent detoxification agent – the antioxidants in 15 lbs of wheatgrass are the equivalent to those in 350 lbs of carrot, lettuce or celery – it must be consumed correctly. And as it is such a powerful cleanser, it may initially cause nausea because it starts up an immediate reaction with toxins and mucus in the stomach.

Begin with one ounce a day with a small amount of water. Once you are accustomed to it, you should stop the water and work up to six ounces of wheatgrass juice a day, at which point your energy levels will be very high. Wheatgrass juice should be also be mixed thoroughly with your saliva before swallowing and drunk, slowly, one hour before meals. It can also be mixed with other juices.

HOW TO GROW WHEATGRASS

Growing your own wheatgrass is probably the easiest way, unless you have an organic store on your doorstep or a good juice bar near your workplace. The seeds can be obtained from organic stores and some health-food stores. One tray will last one person about a week at one shot a day.

--→ Fill a tray with a layer of earth about one inch deep.

--→ Add the seeds and water daily, keeping the tray away from excessive light and temperatures.

--→ Wheatgrass will grow only in fairly warm temperatures so, in winter, it needs to be kept indoors.

--→ After harvesting, new seed must be planted for the next crop, rather like cress.

--→ After about six days the wheatgrass is ready to be cut and juiced. It should be drunk in 1oz shots.

JUICE HEALTH GUIDE

A quick reminder of which vegetables and vegetable mixtures are useful for various everyday ailments. Coconut milk, pomegranate and cranberry are also included for the exceptional benefits that they provide.

Bloating and flatulence: ginger, cumin, fennel, celery

Cleansing liver: carrot, beetroot, beetroot-celery-ginger

Constipation: celery

Detoxification: wheatgrass

Gastric hyperacidity: celery, spinach, carrot

Headaches: celery, carrot-celery-parsley-spinach, coconut milk-carrot

Improving digestion: beetroot, ginger, carrot

Improving immune system: carrot, ginger, garlic, wheatgrass

Kidney (bladder) problems: celery-pomegranate, cranberry

Kidneys: carrot-parsley-asparagus, carrot-parsley, spinach, beetroot-celery-ginger

Overweight, obesity: beet greens-parsley-celery, spinach, celery, lettuce

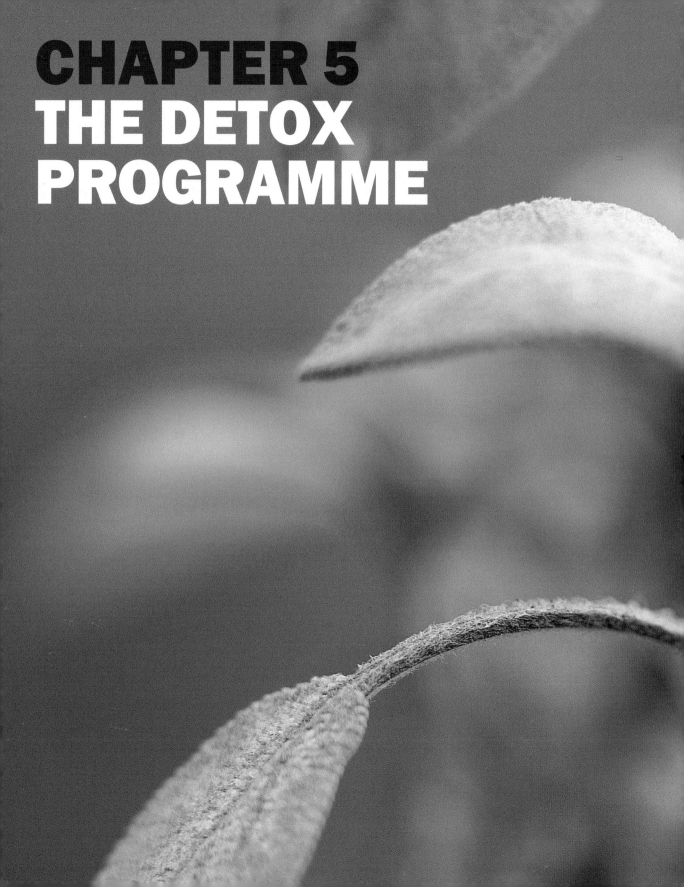

CHAPTER 5
THE DETOX PROGRAMME

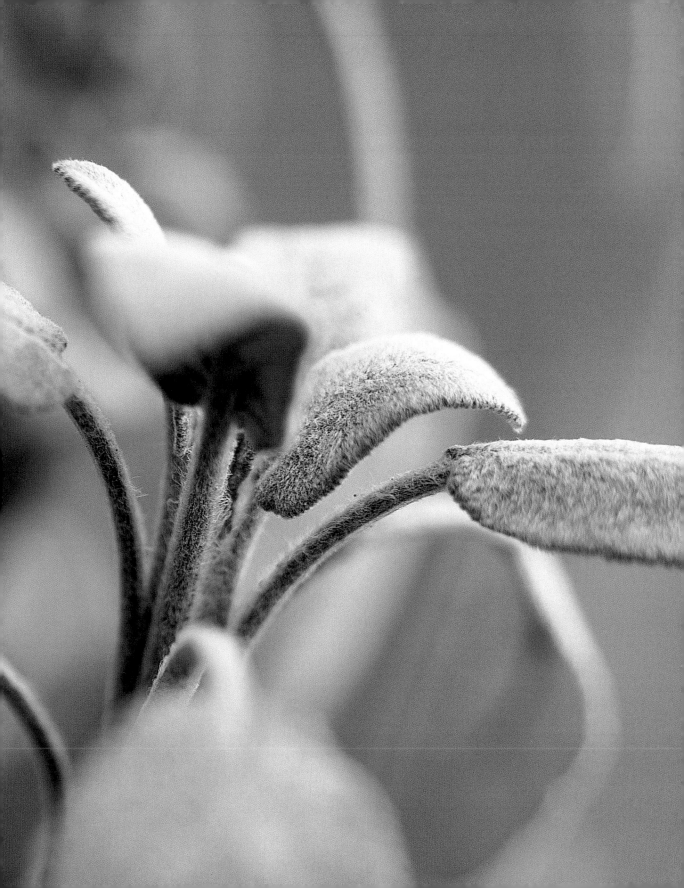

JUST BEFORE YOU GET STARTED ON THE DETOX PROGRAMME, USE THE TONGUE ANALYSIS CHARTS TO ASSESS WHETHER YOU ARE SUFFERING FROM SPECIFIC CONDITIONS AND THE FOLLOWING BODY MASS INDEX FORMULA CHART TO ASSESS WHETHER YOU ARE OVER OR UNDER WEIGHT. THERE IS ALSO A PROGRESS CHART FOR YOU TO RECORD YOUR EXPERIENCES ON THE 21-DAY DETOX PROGRAMME AND CHART YOUR BODY'S CHANGING REACTIONS TO FOOD.

TONGUE ANALYSIS

Using non-invasive methods to diagnose general conditions within the human body has long been part of Eastern medical philosophy. The Chinese, for instance, developed a method of analysing the tongue after noticing that the colourings and indentations displayed by people's tongues matched conditions they were experiencing elsewhere in their bodies. For instance, someone with a poor circulation and suffering from varicose veins would manifest a purple tongue with black spots. Even doctors trained in Western medicine have adopted this practice. We have all been asked to stick out our tongue by our GP, at some point in our lives, so he can look for any abnormalities in its texture, colour and motility that may indicate a problem.

By analysing your own tongue and by checking with the Ayurvedic Profile Chart on page 120, you can learn a lot about your body. Providing you are not suffering any serious condition, you can also learn how to eliminate such ailments as your lethargy and sluggishness by changing your diet.

Tongue diagnoses

A normal tongue is one that is neither too thick nor thin. It is pink in colour all over with a light coating of saliva. There should be no indentations, discolorations, spots, marks or sensitive points. The texture should be smooth and fleshy and it should also be able to move freely.

Tongue description: thin white coating, teeth marks down the sides, pale pink tongue with a few red spots = fatigue, poor appetite, spontaneous sweating, shortness of breath, over-thinking and worrying

Tongue description: thin yellow coating, red surface = feel hot, sweat easily, thirsty, constipated, irritable, bad tempered, skin problems

Tongue description: white greasy coating, swollen tongue = bloated, fullness in chest and abdomen, feel heavy and lethargic

Tongue description: purple surface with black spots = cold limbs, varicose veins, painful legs, headaches, chest pain, liver spots, lack of skin lustre

Tongue description: normal with red tip = stressed, tendency to be depressed and upset, unstable emotional state, prone to pre-menstrual tension

Tongue description: red surface with yellow greasy coating = skin problems, urinary infections, clammy skin, angry and uncomfortable

Tongue description: pale pink swollen surface, thick white coating = feels cold easily, always needs warmth, pale complexion, back pain, tendency to panic, emotionally low, potentially impotent, infertile

Tongue description: red surface with cracks, little or no coating = prone to hot flushes, sweats at night, insomnia, irritable, ringing in the ears, irregular menstrual cycle

Tongue description: pale surface, little or no coating = dizziness, fatigue, palpitations, poor memory, insomnia, irregular periods

BODY MASS INDEX FORMULA

The Body Mass Index can be used to indicate whether you are underweight, of normal weight, overweight or obese. BMI is an objective scientific measure that uses your height and weight to calculate your body mass. I prefer this as a means of weight measurement, as it is more important to strive for a normal BMI than achieve a certain weight (which may not be one that's healthy for you). You can calculate your BMI by dividing your weight in kilograms by the square of your height in metres (BMI=kg/m^2), or by using a BMI calculator which is available on several websites.

BMI = a person's weight in kilograms divided by height in metres squared.

BMI metric formula
BMI = Weight [in kilos] divided by
(Height [in metres] X Height [in metres])
or:

BMI Pounds/Inches Formula
BMI = Weight [in pounds] x 704.5 divided by (Height [in inches] x Height [in inches])

BMI examples
You are 63 inches in height.
Your weight is 135 pounds.
Your Body Mass Index is 24. (normal weight)

You are 66 inches in height.
Your weight is 161 pounds.
Your Body Mass Index is 26. (overweight)

You are 64 inches in height.
Your weight is 174 pounds.
Your Body Mass Index is 30. (obese)

BMI results
18.5 or less = underweight
18.5 – 24.9 = normal weight
25 – 29.9 = overweight
30 – 34.9 = obese
35 – 39 = very obese
40 plus = dangerously obese

BODY MASS INDEX CHART

Height	Weight in Pounds																					
58"	91	96	100	105	110	115	119	124	129	134	138	143	148	153	158	162	167	172	177	181	186	191
59"	94	99	104	109	114	119	124	128	133	138	143	148	153	158	163	168	173	178	183	188	193	198
60"	97	102	107	112	118	123	128	133	138	143	148	153	158	163	168	174	179	184	189	194	199	204
61"	100	106	111	116	122	127	132	137	143	148	153	158	164	169	174	180	185	190	195	201	206	211
62"	104	109	115	120	126	131	136	142	147	153	158	164	169	175	180	186	191	196	202	207	213	218
63"	107	113	118	124	130	135	141	146	152	158	163	169	175	180	186	191	197	203	208	214	220	225
64"	110	116	122	128	134	140	145	151	157	163	169	174	180	186	192	197	204	209	215	221	227	232
65"	114	120	126	132	138	144	150	156	162	168	174	180	186	192	198	204	210	216	222	228	234	240
66"	118	124	130	136	142	148	155	161	167	173	179	186	192	198	204	210	216	223	229	235	241	247
67"	121	127	134	140	146	153	159	166	172	178	185	191	198	204	211	217	223	230	236	242	249	255
68"	125	131	138	144	151	158	164	171	177	184	190	197	203	210	216	223	230	236	243	249	256	262
69"	128	135	142	149	155	162	169	176	182	189	196	203	209	216	223	230	236	243	250	257	263	270
70"	132	139	146	153	160	167	174	181	188	195	202	209	216	222	229	236	243	250	257	264	271	278
71"	136	143	150	157	165	172	179	186	193	200	208	215	222	229	236	243	250	257	265	272	279	286
72"	140	147	154	162	169	177	184	191	199	206	213	221	228	235	242	250	257	265	272	279	287	294
73"	144	151	159	166	174	182	189	197	204	212	219	227	235	242	250	257	265	272	280	288	295	302
74"	148	155	163	171	179	186	194	202	210	218	225	233	241	249	256	264	272	280	287	295	303	311
BMI	19	20	21	22	23	24	25	26	27	28	29	30	31	32	33	34	35	36	37	38	39	40

PROGRESS CHART

Score points from 1 to 5 and complete
the chart at the beginning of each week
of the Detox Programme.

1 = very frequent/severe symptoms
2 = regular/bad symptoms
3 = fairly regular/tolerable symptoms
4 = infrequent/manageable symptoms
5 = rare/minor symptoms

	Week One	Week Two	Week Three
Bloating	☐	☐	☐
BMI score	☐	☐	☐
Constipation	☐	☐	☐
Energy levels	3	☐	☐
Exercise (frequency)	☐	☐	☐
Headaches	2	☐	☐
Heartburn	–	☐	☐
Indigestion	–	☐	☐
Insomnia	4	☐	☐
Lethargy	☐	☐	☐
Menopausal hot flushes	–	☐	☐
Mental clarity	☐	☐	☐
Mood swings	–	☐	☐
Motivation/will-power	☐	☐	☐
Self-confidence	☐	☐	☐
Skin problems	☐	☐	☐
Sugar cravings	4	☐	☐

Are you embarking on this Detox Programme because you want to lose weight? Have more energy? Feel less tired? Less bloated? Less constipated? Do you want to recapture all your pre-life-stressed attractiveness? Have lovelier skin? Glossier hair? Radiant self-confidence?

As I explained in the Introduction, my interest in diet and nutrition started years ago when I was treating ballet dancers. They had such a poor perception of themselves that they would eat tissue paper, smoke cigarettes and drink coca cola rather than have a piece of grilled chicken because they thought that any food would make them fat. As a result of their appalling diet, they had no energy and even less strength and they were constantly suffering from sprained ankles, strained muscles, pulled tendons and stress fractures. I encouraged them to eat healthily and to nurture themselves more and, as a result, they began to feel stronger and to dance better. They were less tired, were able to dance for longer and didn't suffer so many injuries. They were confidant, healthier and, most of, all happier.

It is useful to know your motivations for doing this Detox Programme because then you can start to think ahead and decide where you would like to go from here. Maybe you want to improve your self-confidence and self-esteem in order to improve your job prospects. Maybe you want to take up a certain sport or activity, or become more knowledgeable about nutrition, so you can cook healthier meals for you and your family.

Why not think about where you would like to see yourself not only in three weeks time but also, perhaps, in six months, one year – or even five. A fundamental point of my Detox is longevity. This is not just a quick fix; it's a way of changing the whole way you eat which will have an enormous effect on your health and whole way of life.

AT-A-GLANCE FOOD CHART

FOODS TO AVOID OR REDUCE

- Acidic drinks e.g. orange juice, grapefruit juice, apple juice
- Alcohol especially wine, champagne, beer
- All (especially citrus) fruit/fruit juices (except ripe bananas)
- Baked beans, pizza, processed foods, fried and spicy foods
- Low-fat yoghurts and reduced-fat foods (usually loaded with sugar, carbohydrates and chemicals)
- Bread/wheat and gluten products, pasta
- Dairy foods (cheese, milk and butter)
- Fizzy drinks, tonic water and carbonated flavoured waters
- Nuts (except pine nuts and seeds)
- Potatoes, aubergines, mushrooms, cucumbers, courgettes, tomatoes, peppers, avocados
- Red meat – lamb, beef, pork, ham, sausages
- Shellfish – prawns, mussels, crab, lobster, shrimps
- Sugar and chocolates, cakes, biscuits, croissants, muffins
- Tea/coffee (except green tea and herbal teas e.g. camomile/rosehip/peppermint)
- Tomato ketchup, vinegar, mustard, sauces, chutneys
- Yeast and yeast products (check the labels on food products e.g. soy sauce, pickles, Marmite)

FOODS TO INCREASE

- Brown rice
- Buffalo mozzarella (occasionally as a cheese alternative)
- Dark green vegetables (except avocados which are acidic so should be eaten in moderation)
- Eggs (but not more than 3–4 times per week)
- Fish (especially oily fish such as sardines, but not shellfish, tuna or swordfish)
- Freshly-made vegetable juices
- Freshly-made vegetable soups
- Gluten-free oatmeal made with rice milk or water
- Gluten-free/wheat-free breads
- Gluten-free/wheat-free cereals
- Goats' cheese, ricotta, cottage cheese
- Honey
- Live yoghurt
- Olive oil
- Pulses/lentils/chick peas
- Salads (excluding tomatoes and peppers) and steamed vegetables
- Soya and tofu products
- Soya milk, rice milk, goats milk
- White meat – chicken, turkey
- NOTE: Seasonings, salt/pepper are allowed in moderation

DEALING WITH TEMPTATIONS

It is a sad fact of life that we don't become addicted to those foods that are good for us but only to foods that are potentially toxic and which generate chemical imbalances and dysfunctions within the body.

At the start of your three-week detox, it may seem almost impossible to stay away from alcohol, saturated fats, sugars, cakes and chocolates. But three weeks isn't really a long time. All you need is a little will power and determination, in the first phase, to avoid the things you know are bad for you. Use the Conquering Cravings chart to note how your tastes start to switch to far more nutritious foods, and how items that you previously couldn't live without now have little or no hold over you.

ANALYSING YOUR CRAVINGS

One important goal, on the Detox, is reprogramming your body to stem its greed in demanding an immediate (addictive) 'hit' of sugar and salt, or a stimulant such as caffeine or alcohol, and settle for receiving a gradual release (of whatever you currently require) from healthier foods such as a gluten/wheat-free muffin, honey, yoghurt, carrots for sugar, corn chips or slightly salted seeds and nuts for salt, and plain fresh filtered water if you need a boost. In other words you are weaning yourself off those foods that are bad for you and replacing them with ones that are good.

Another very important thing is to be able to distinguish between a healthy and unhealthy craving. If you experience thirst, then quench it with pure filtered water rather than a glass of milk or a fizzy drink. The body's tissues can only absorb essential minerals and nutrients in water, so the reason why you feel thirsty is probably because the body is telling you that it is dehydrated and needs more water to nourish the tissues.

If you feel tired, especially after exercise, you may need to replace some of the salt the body has lost which is why I recommend washing down some slightly salty seeds or chopped nuts (unless you are nut-allergic) with lots of fresh water. Corn chips can also satisfy a salt craving without loading the body with acid from the potatoes that are used to make crisps. If you have a sudden urge for a sugary taste, then have a banana or a herbal tea with honey which have more nutrients and vitamins than a bar of chocolate. If you crave a bitter taste, this may well be your body telling you it requires some vitamin C, so drink a glass of hot water with a slice of lemon rather than some acidic orange juice.

What you are aiming to do is get your body off the roller coaster of having peaks and troughs of blood sugar and salt levels. You are trying to achieve balance, remember, so better a slow rise and wane than sudden highs and lows. This is why by feeding your body foods that gradually release the sugar or salt you desire, you will satisfy your cravings in a better way and, in time, get your body used to having less sugar and salt. As a result, you will soon no longer experience cravings at all.

CONQUERING CRAVINGS

Tick the foods you most crave during Week One in column one, Week Two in column two, and so on, and similarly mark the foods you least crave with a cross. See for yourself how your body's demands change over the course of the Detox.

Complete the Conquering Cravings chart at the end of each of the three weeks of the Detox to gauge how effective you are becoming at combating your cravings. You will notice that the foods you crave in Week One will be different to those you crave in Weeks Two and Three. This is because you are re-educating your palate to reject the extreme tastes of the very sugary (cakes and chocolates) and the very salty (crisps).

Foods	Week One	Week Two	Week Three
Alcohol	☐	☐	☐
Bread	☐	☐	☐
Cakes	☐	☐	☐
Cheese	☐	☐	☐
Chocolate	☐	☐	☐
Cigarettes	☐	☐	☐
Coffee/Tea	☐	☐	☐
Crisps	☐	☐	☐
Fatty foods	☐	☐	☐
Fried foods	☐	☐	☐
Fruit	☐	☐	☐
Junk foods	☐	☐	☐
Orange juice	☐	☐	☐
Pasta	☐	☐	☐
Potatoes	☐	☐	☐
Red meat	☐	☐	☐
Sugar	☐	☐	☐
Water	☐	☐	☐

MOMENTS OF WEAKNESS

Life is for living and there will always be social events and activities that bring you face to face with foods that you should be avoiding. That is why, with my Detox Programme, all is not lost if you are 'forced' to give in to temptation. If you are going to be naughty, it is not the end of the world. You are not suddenly going to revert back to square one and undo all the good you have done. Succumbing to a cheese straw and a glass of sherry at the chairman's cocktail party isn't going to wreck all your hard work. Hopefully, after the three weeks of Detox training you'll be able to control your 'naughtier' days or plan them so they are not going to stretch into naughty weeks.

My sweet-toothed patients find the hardest things to avoid are delicious desserts. When the option of a dessert arises, think about the nutritional content of what you are eating or the choice you have on a menu. How much nutritional content are you going to derive from a slice of chocolate gateau, or a crème caramel? Even though it is extraordinarily tasty and tempting, once you have taken that mouthful you will only feel guilty and unhappy when you discover later that you have piled on those lost few pounds.

If you're going to be naughty, in terms of dessert, I recommend having a fruit salad, or maybe a sorbet. The alternative is to cheat by having a spoonful of everybody else's, rather than ordering one of your own. If you're desperate for a quick fix, remember that a chromium supplement will help your body maintain balanced blood sugar levels by metabolising your fat (which is more desirable if you are seeking to lose some weight).

When it comes to wine, try to make sure that it is very good quality and drink a glass of water for each glass of wine you consume. This will dilute its alcoholic effect and make it easier for the liver to neutralise. However, it would be far better to avoid wine for these three weeks – and whisky and beer. These are all fermented drinks that allow yeast growth in the gut which makes it congested and unhealthy (and can lead to candida).

If you cannot resist alcohol during the Maintenance Programme, the best alternatives are unfermented alcohols such as gin or vodka. If you are going to have vodka, avoid having tonic water with it (which is full of chemicals) and opt instead for a plain vodka martini, or one with watermelon, kiwi, pomegranate juice or sugar-free cranberry. Cranberries are particularly recommended for people who suffer from cystitis because they neutralise acidity in the kidneys and the bladder.

GOING STRAIGHT AGAIN

Even if you have a history of becoming racked with guilt and depression every time you 'cheat' on a diet, I implore you not to be too hard on yourself during my Detox Programme. Most diets make you feel that you have negated all the good work you have done if you give in to temptation even once. That is not the case with my Holistic Detox Programme.

There is no question that it will take a while to persuade your palate that it doesn't need refined sugars, so the odd lapse is forgivable. But when I say 'odd' I mean 'occasional' and not 'frequent'. One chocolate square is OK – an entire bar is not. One chocolate square every day is bearable but a box of chocolates or biscuits is hopeless.

Feeding your craving will only make it worse. Finding alternatives will not only take away the need to cheat but possibly put your body into shock if you do cheat. If you have not eaten refined sugars if only for a week, and then succumb to a biscuit or slice of cake, you may suffer a headache or feel bloated. You had just got your body back onto a healthy, even keel, and used to having a low blood-sugar level, and then you suddenly gave it a major hit, sending that level sky high. Even so, it is not the end of the world if this happens. Just resume your intention to establish – for yourself – the discipline of eating nutritional foods, and keep reminding yourself that foods with low nutritional value are only feeding the old cravings and not the new, Detoxed you.

CHANGING YOUR PALATE

During the Detox Programme (providing you stick to the menus and don't cheat much), you will discover that your palate will change. If you avoid the no-nos such as bread, chocolate and alcohol, you will find – hard as it may be to believe – that after a while you won't actually like the taste of bread any more. Neither will you enjoy chocolate so much, nor sugar, and you may actually wince when you have a sip of orange juice or wine because it has come to taste quite acidic and coffee will just taste bitter. This is the pay-off for all the work you'll have been doing to alter the pH balance in your body from acid to alkaline. In so doing, you've been weaning your taste buds off addictive and toxic foods. You are programming them to reject the taste of foods that they are learning to recognise as 'bad'!

NEW FOOD PATTERNS

This Detox is designed to encourage you to change your dietary habits and also the way you shop, prepare foods and consume them. I recommend, for example, that you chew each mouthful at least eight to ten times to make sure that the food matter is broken down into the smallest possible size. The smaller it is, the easier it is for you to digest it and your body to derive from it the maximum amount of nutrients. This applies particularly to vegetables because, as you chew them, you are breaking down the fibrous sheaths in which all the nutrients are stored so that all the goodness can be released. Similarly, in chewing meat you are actually tenderising it – which makes life a lot easier for your stomach.

In the mornings, I recommend waking up with a slice of lemon in a glass of warm water – sipped slowly. Water not only acts as a cleansing tonic, flushing toxins from the kidneys, but it is a non-stimulant and so allows the body's own natural stimulants to kick-start your day. Do make it a firm habit; apart from benefiting you enormously, it's the first step towards lessening those caffeine cravings.

Throughout the day, instead of caffeinated drinks, try and drink two litres of filtered water, or a glass every hour, if that's easier– setting an alarm on your watch or phone to remind you. Resist adding cordials or juices; these only give your body yet another detoxifying job to do.

MEALTIMES

As busy as you might be, at mealtimes it is worth taking the time to sit where you can focus on what you're eating, even at work. You will never see a Frenchman eat a sandwich at his desk – and it is no coincidence that the French suffer fewer incidences of heart disease, obesity and certain cancers than we do. I maintain that this is because, in France, mealtimes are sacred occasions. At lunchtime, most schoolchildren and workers still return home to sit with their families around the table for a nutritious meal. No matter how busy you are, try and make a pact with yourself not to eat at your desk. Better to sit with a salad in the corner of the canteen than chew on a chicken leg over your keyboard.

For the purposes of the Holistic Detox, sitting round the table with the family for breakfast or evening meals can be enormously valuable for a variety of reasons, not least in finding out what your children have been up to. It is also an excellent time for families to re-bond, re-learn the art of conversation and keep the lines of communication open, even if they may sometimes be strained.

With so many demands on our time, there are not many opportunities in the day when we can all get together without distractions to catch up on each other's lives. Mealtimes are one of the few opportunities when this can happen. If you are a parent, it also allows you to keep a check on what your children are eating. Now you are doing the Detox, you will also be aware of just how many chemicals are contained in those ready-made dinners that the kids have been re-heating in the microwave. It is also quite possible for you to adapt your own delicious healthy supper of grilled chicken and vegetables into something appetising for your children – just by adding a few potatoes, perhaps, or a freshly-made tomato sauce. This is an opportunity to rethink mealtimes, not as an irritating interruption to your busy schedule, but as quality time with your loved ones. Take time to savour each mouthful and chew your food as much as possible. Your body will appreciate it – particularly if it isn't forced to sit slouched in front of the television! Eating slowly will also fill you up faster so you will eat smaller portions.

DRINK JUST A LITTLE DURING MEALS

Taking too much fluid while eating can dilute your vital digestive enzymes. I recommend sipping water (served at room temperature) during meals and then perhaps drinking half an hour after you have finished. This will maintain a wonderfully fluid medium through which your nutrients can be digested and absorbed. Being dehydrated doesn't just affect your absorption of toxins, it also limits the amount of nutrients you can ingest. This is because nutrients are more easily absorbed within a watery environment. Being dehydrated will also slow down your digestive process thereby encouraging your food to get stuck and start putrefying before it's been expelled.

MEALS FOR ONE

Eating for one should be an equally enriching experience. Even when you are alone, allow yourself time to enjoy your food. The reason you may tend to rush your meals, or eat in front of the television, is perhaps because you are not that interested in what you are eating. After all, you have probably eaten the meal a thousand times before, so it no longer holds any interest or surprises.

By trying new foods and experimenting with menus, you will make the experience of mealtimes more enjoyable and interesting. They can give you ideas for your next dinner party. You can avoid the temptation of a take-away or pre-prepared meal by choosing something quick and easy such as steamed fish and vegetables or grilled chicken flavoured with some exotic spices and herbs (see the Recipes section at the back of the book). Choose foods that are as fresh as possible because they will have more flavour. Remember to savour each mouthful and chew it eight to ten times. Eating slowly allows the body to digest manageable amounts of food rather than having to process large amounts all at once, so you will feel full before you have eaten your last mouthful. Try not to wolf down your meal in ten minutes flat – make an occasion if it. Nurture yourself and your body. Even if I am eating alone, I never take a phone call during mealtimes.

HOSTING A DETOX DINNER PARTY

Use your imagination when hosting dinner parties. Try not to feel daunted, there really are a host of options and, with a little planning, there's no reason for your guests to feel deprived. Use the recipes at the back of the book for inspiration and enjoy getting creative. For example, you could start with a small green salad on a bed of steamed asparagus drizzled with extra virgin olive oil and some sea salt and chopped mint.

Next, serve steamed spinach, broccoli, mange tout and some red cabbage with some steamed salmon or any fish garnished with parsley, lemon slices, and seasonal herbs such as dill, or perhaps roast a chicken that you have marinated in yoghurt with some mint, coriander or dill. For dessert, serve a frozen banana special made from blended banana and soya yoghurt, sweetened with molasses or honey, flavoured with a touch of cardamom, sprinkled with chopped banana pieces and garnished with some fresh mint.

Other than still water, the drinks could be vodka or gin martinis with some freshly squeezed watermelon, pomegranate or even banana juice! There are lots more recipes in the Recipe section that you can adapt to give your friends some exotic *je ne sais quoi* without them ever realising that they're eating a Detox dinner. I promise they will come back for more.

EATING OUT DURING THE DETOX

Remember the three-week Detox Plan is not about feeling deprived but about discovering new foods, so don't feel you have to hide yourself away for the duration.

Obviously, when you eat out, there are certain things you cannot control. However, if everything on the menu is immersed in butter, ask if they can grill you some chicken or fish. Ask them, too, if they add any gluten to their dishes.

In an Italian restaurant, for example, choose the Dover sole with steamed greens. If you are dining at Pizza Express, choose the salad nicoise; the pasta will be a no-no, I am afraid, as will be the dough balls and garlic bread but there will always be an alternative. In a Thai restaurant, try the satay chicken, or the rice noodles with vegetables, with a clear soup. Be sure it's not too spicy otherwise you may get hyperacidity. The choices are numerous if only you look at the menu and don't automatically plump for all the usual favourites which have, in the past, made you feel bloated, sluggish and heavy.

LIVER FLUSH

I recommend making yourself a liver flush every week during the three-week Programme and drinking it at a time when you can sit and relax quietly for a couple of hours afterwards. My special recipe improves liver function by stimulating the elimination of toxins and waste products from the body, thereby acting as a fast track to detox success. It also helps purify the blood and lymphatic system.

Ingredients:
Grapefruit, lemon, garlic, ginger root, extra-virgin olive oil.

Method:
1. Take about 300ml of freshly squeezed grapefruit and lemon juice and dilute this with 200ml of filtered water.
2. Grate 1 or 2 cloves of fresh garlic and a small piece of ginger root and, using a garlic press, squeeze this juice into the fruit juice mixture. Garlic and ginger are liver cleansing and protective. Garlic contains sulphur compounds that the liver needs for its detoxification enzymes.
3. Add 2tbs of cold-pressed extra-virgin olive oil and mix with the juice in a blender. Drink.
4. Follow this with 2 cups of cleansing herbal teas made from 3–4 herbs. The ones I recommend are fennel, dandelion root, fenugreek, peppermint, chickweed, nettle and parsley.

Liver-flush routine
I suggest drinking the liver flush in the morning after a brisk walk (20 minutes minimum) and followed by some deep breathing. For this, sit cross-legged. Take long deep breaths, inhaling through the nose and exhaling through the mouth 20 times. Focus on the inhalation and exhalation, taking your time to fill your lungs and then exhaling even more slowly. This is a fantastic stress-busting exercise. You will feel instantly calmer afterwards. (You can do this breathing exercise anywhere any time.) It is best to close your eyes so you can focus more easily. Try to keep your back straight while you expand your chest. After your deep breaths, lie down and relax for about 2 hours. Make sure, during the day, that you drink about 2 litres of water.

THE DETOX PROGRAMME
WEEK ONE

WAKING UP: Boil a kettle with filtered water and pour into a cup. Pop in a slice of lemon, leave to cool to drinking temperature and sip slowly. If you are taking chromium, selenium, digest aid, or liver-cleanse supplements, this is a good time to take them. Obviously you do not have to take any supplements during the Detox, but many patients find they achieve better results more quickly if they do.

Take a moment to examine your tongue. Its condition can tell you a huge amount about your health. Examine it properly and note the results.

Complete your Progress Chart, your Body Mass Index and your Conquering Cravings Chart. By keeping these results in an obvious place – such as stuck to the fridge door – you can monitor your progress throughout the Detox. I suggest you do these three tests at the beginning of each week, rather than every day.

BREAKFAST: Mix a bowl of gluten-free/wheat-free muesli with either rice or soya milk. Do not be tempted to add sugar but, instead, add a chopped banana. Another option is to make scrambled eggs by mixing two eggs with no butter but with either rice or soya milk and place them on a slice of toasted gluten-free/wheat-free bread. Alternatively, fill a teacup with either Greek or natural live yoghurt and mix with a little organic honey. A glass of freshly-squeezed vegetable juice is a brilliant start to the day. See pages 81–3 for ideas.

MID-MORNING SNACK: Peel and chop two or three large organic carrots into sticks, add some raw bok choi, cauliflower florets and mange tout and place in a plastic food bag. These make delicious snacks which you can keep in your handbag or car and eat throughout the day – or when you get a sugar craving. Don't forget to drink plenty of water, too; sometimes that, alone, can satisfy sugar cravings – or a herbal tea with a little honey.

LUNCH: There are lots of healthy and nutritious lunch and dinner recipes at the back of this book ranging from delicious vegetable soups to exciting chicken, fish and vegetarian dishes. Explore and enjoy. For the three-week period, taking a packed lunch to work is preferable – unless your office canteen serves freshly made salads, homemade vegetable stir fries and soups. If not, take your own homemade chicken or vegetable soup in a flask, a salad or any of the suggestions in the Recipe section. Always make sure you drink plenty of water and if you're taking supplements take them at that time.

If you have to dine out at lunchtime, ask the waiter if the chef can grill you some fish or chicken or prepare a delicious stir-fry of fresh vegetables. Most restaurants can manage simple off-menu dishes. If you have an hour for lunch, but don't need all that time to eat, then go for a brisk walk for 20 minutes (weather permitting). Also explore the company's sporting facilities. Many offices have gymnasiums with showers, or special discounted deals with local fitness centres.

TEA: If you do feel peckish around mid-afternoon, then opt for a herbal tea (green tea is refreshing) and, perhaps, a gluten-free/wheat-free biscuit – but watch out, they are calorific. If you have a fridge at work, keep some hummus or homemade guacamole in there, and dip into them with some rice crackers as a snack.

Try to resist the boxes of chocolates and birthday cakes that do the rounds in offices, but don't be too virtuous. What you eat is your own business. I would recommend not alerting all and sundry to the fact that you have embarked on a life-changing Detox Plan – unless you believe your colleagues will be supportive. From my experience, most people will want to test your resolve, place temptation in your path – and watch you fail! Better to get on with it quietly so that it does not become the whole focus of your life. People will realise soon enough what you are up to when they notice how fantastic you are looking, how much energy you have and how slim you are.

SUPPER: Whether you live alone, or with a loved one and/or family, anyone with whom you have a close relationship will have to be involved with your Plan. So, if you can tempt your family or friends round to your dinner table for supper, this would not just benefit you in re-affirming relations with them but also benefit them nutritionally, whether you live with an unreasonable parent, irascible teenager, stressed-out partner or hyper-active toddler. No matter how old we are, we can all benefit from a diet free of refined sugars, carbohydrates, additives, stimulants and chemicals. So get people in your life on board, even if it is only for one meal a day.

BEDTIME: It may be barely 24 hours since you started the Detox but, if you have stuck to my food advice, you could be feeling the benefits already. If the end of the day finds you stressed and uptight, relax with some calming camomile or peppermint tea. For some of you, it will be good, at bedtime, to take a detoxing remedy which will

work overnight and help rid the body of any congested waste matter and toxins.

Repeat this Detox Diet for the next seven days, varying recipes and referring to the Food Charts for reminders of what you can and can't eat. Don't forget the liver flush – this will stimulate your metabolism to work more efficiently and speed you on your way to success.

You may find it useful to keep a journal of how you're feeling as you detox. Many people find the end of the day a good time to record their thoughts and feelings.

FIVE TOP DETOXING TIPS
1. Start the day with a glass of warm water with a little fresh lemon juice squeezed in to flush the kidneys.
2. Chew your food at least 8–12 times, and eat slowly.
3. Sip water during meals and then drink water about half an hour after eating.
4. Have smaller meals more times a day.
5. Drink about 1–2 litres of water or herbal teas daily.
Warning: You may feel headaches, increased tiredness and nausea for the first few days. This is the Detox process beginning. If you are concerned about these symptoms, stop the Detox and seek advice from your doctor.
Please take herbal teas with some honey every two to three hours until the symptoms subside.

THE DETOX PROGRAMME
WEEK TWO

WAKING UP: While you should still stick to your hot water-and-lemon early-morning tonic, you can alternate this with some herbal teas – ensuring they are caffeine free. Green tea is also excellent in the morning for its refreshing and antioxidant characteristics; although it does contain some caffeine, the levels are substantially lower than in coffee or other teas.

Some companies produce teas which are just what you need for the Detox (for websites, see the Directory). Twinings offer a green-tea blend of both black and green teas that come from the same plant, *Camellia sinensis*, and are a rich source of antioxidants. Jacksons of Piccadilly make an organic blend of green tea and camomile that is very calming and relaxing and is probably best taken at the end of the day to unwind, or in the morning if you have had a restless night. Clearspring produce an organic Japanese Sencha green tea that comes in leaves rather than tea bags. Sencha is used by Zen monks to promote mental clarity and calmness during prolonged meditations. Clipper manufacture a delicious Ayurvedic Detox Infusion that is an organic blend of rosemary, ginger, oregano, turmeric, aloe vera and lime.

At the beginning of the second week, take time to check your Progress Chart as well as your BMI, Tongue Analysis and Conquering Cravings chart. Compare your results with the ones you took a week ago and note any changes. Ideally you should be scoring higher numbers in your Progress Chart than last week. Don't worry if you aren't – people progress at different rates. If there are no changes yet, don't get despondent. The important thing is that there soon will be.

BREAKFAST: Follow the general pattern of Week One, alternating with vegetable juices, gluten-free oatmeal made with rice milk or water, banana, yoghurt with honey, and/or boiled eggs with gluten-free toasted soldiers.

Instead of driving to work/taking the bus/train, try and walk some of the distance, or cycle if it is not too dangerous. If this is going to mean getting up half an hour earlier to walk for 20 minutes– it's worth it, I promise. It will set your body and mind up for the day. Exercise not only increases your metabolic rate but it stimulates the brain, too. What's more, that increased rate will remain throughout the day, which will boost your chance of losing weight, and enhance your energy levels.

MID-MORNING SNACK: Continue with your healthy option of freshly chopped carrot sticks, bok choi and cauliflower. These are packed with nutrients and fibre to fill the gap.

LUNCH: As a challenge, try to arrange to have lunch with a colleague, relative or friend with whom you have some unfinished business or a problem to resolve. See how the environment of a meal can break down barriers and help sort out a relationship problem or misunderstanding which has been nagging you. While you will know what you should and should not eat by now, try not to make the actual food the focus of the meal. Choose carefully from the menu (refer to page 110 for some tips) but take the time to address the more emotional aspects of the 21–Day Detox. If you're experiencing negative emotions such as anger or bitterness, this can have a serious effect on your health, triggering headaches, abdominal pains, high blood pressure and anxiety.

TEA: This is usually the time in many people's day when they have a slump in energy levels. This may be due to a small drop in blood supply to the brain as your body is busy digesting the nutrients from lunch. Go for the healthy option, some seeds and nuts with filtered water and feel yourself revive.

DINNER: Refer to the Recipe chapter for inspiration if you are cooking for yourself or your family. Or use the 21-Day Detox as the incentive to try out new activities and ways of eating out. Exercise is a crucial component of the programme, so try a new sport or take a dance class or a yoga course. If you can share your new pastime with a friend and follow it up with a light supper and a good chat, so much the better. This would be a great night out – without any unpleasant side-effects, and will relax you hugely because of the endorphins which are released through exercise. Endorphins are neurotransmitters that have pain-relieving properties similar to morphine and can produce sensations of ecstasy.

BED-TIME: You will be more than ready for your night-cap after spending an exhilarating evening doing something healthy and different – so pop the kettle on and make a camomile tea, or sip on a glass of filtered water. If you have decided to include any extra detoxing supplements (or senna) in the Programme, don't forget to take them before it gets too late. Many of them need a good eight hours in which to work. You should, by now, be enjoying an uninterrupted night's sleep (unless you suffer from insomnia or have a young baby) and be waking up refreshed, exhilarated and ready to start the day.

Repeat for the next seven days, making sure you are exercising at least three times a week – more if you can manage it. Remember the liver flush, too, which will help cleanse your liver and purify your blood thus boosting your energy levels.

THE DETOX PROGRAMME
WEEK THREE

Start the week with the satisfaction of a Chart Check. The rewards of your commitment will be there to see. By sticking to the Programme, you are scoring higher marks in your Progress Chart, your BMI is on the wane, your Cravings are disappearing and the Tongue Analysis section also indicates that your health is improving. If no one has commented on how great you are looking, they will in a few days time. They won't fail to notice the shrinkage either – aren't your clothes feeling a little looser, aren't you less bloated, less tired?

WAKING UP: Think about incorporating some light exercise at the beginning of your day, after your cup of hot water with lemon and your supplements. It's a great way to stimulate your metabolism, boost vitality and prepare you for the day ahead. Even though you are stronger later in the day when your muscles have woken up, the body burns more calories when you exercise in the morning, so that is the best time for any energetic physical activity.

BREAKFAST: As with Week Two, choose from a selection of gluten-free cereal, rice milk, live yoghurt with honey, and gluten-free/wheat-free bread. If you are feeling more adventurous, you could make yourself some kedgeree with brown rice and flaked salmon, or scrambled eggs and smoked salmon. Don't forget the variety of juices you can have too (see Recipe section).

MID-MORNING: You should have a good early-morning routine going, now, of chopping carrots and other raw vegetables for mid-morning nibbles – or preparing your flask of vegetable juice or herbal tea.

LUNCH: If you have been adventurous you will have been experimenting with the various recipes at the back of the book and also trying out new foods you may not have tried before such as tofu, soya, pulses and lentils. You may also have booked yourself into a yoga or pilates class during your lunch hour, which is an excellent way to de-stress if you have a pressurised job or family. Be careful not to skip meals, though. If you do your blood sugar levels will go haywire which will increase your cravings and the temptation to lunge for that chocolate bar and/or biscuit.

TEA: A banana's a good choice if you feel peckish in the afternoon. They're also an effective pick-you-up if your energy levels wane. For severe nagging cravings, there's the gluten-free shortbread or muffin, but don't reach for these calorie-loaded snacks too often.

SUPPER: Salmon or chicken is a good choice for a light meal, if supper is going to be late. Take care not to eat too late, though, or your body won't have time to digest your food. And while I do not recommend eating leftovers (particularly vegetables as they tend to be less nutritious), I do make an exception for chicken and salmon which are just as delicious, cold, the following day. Make a mental note, now, to serve your own portions on a slightly smaller plate. This will stop you from gorging and over-eating. Also, don't cook too much or you may be tempted to finish it all up.

BED-TIME: Always take a large glass of water to bed, which you can sip during the night if you feel thirsty. This will help to keep your bowels regular and prevent constipation. Take a hot cup of camomile tea if you need a relaxing tonic. (This is particularly good too for any detox or senna capsules you might be taking to de-congest your digestive tract.)

BED-TIME MEDITATION EXERCISES: This week I am going to introduce some gentle meditation exercises which will help relax you if you've had a stressful day, and help you sleep better if you have been experiencing disturbed nights. Meditation, which I talk about in more detail in Chapter 8, has been shown to have therapeutic benefits in relieving illness and stress, lowering blood pressure and enhancing the immune system as well as calming the mind.

I am not going to ask you to assume the lotus position (the classic meditation pose). Just sit so you are comfortable – cross-legged is often best, with your hands gently resting on your thighs. Close your eyes and completely relax your body from head to toe, and then start breathing gently and slowly. Think about inhaling energy – and exhaling stress. Your thoughts may wander, but try and harness them to your breathing, focussing anew on each inhalation and each exhalation, and evenly releasing the tension through your breath. When you feel completely relaxed, slowly open your eyes and then remain still. Then, after a few more minutes, make your way to your bed (if you are not in it already) for a good night's sleep. If you can, repeat this exercise each evening to detox the mind of the stresses and tensions of the day.

Also refer to my Visualisation Exercises in Chapter 8 as a relaxation tonic.

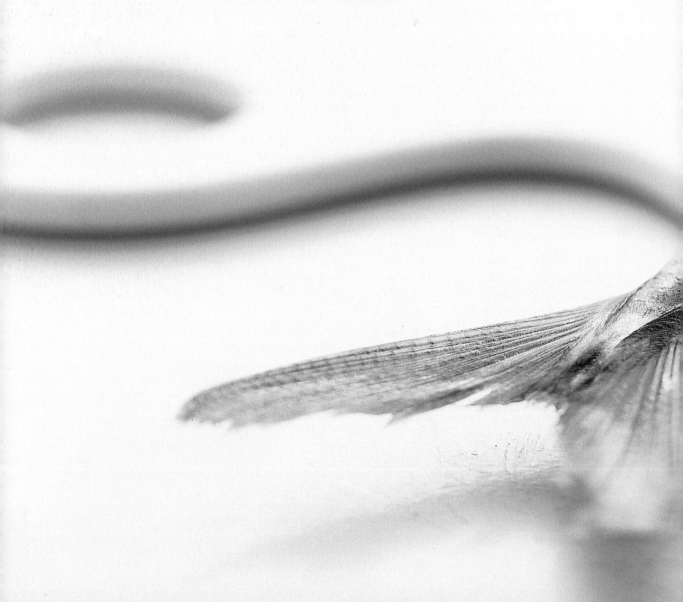

CHAPTER 6
THE MAINTENANCE PROGRAMME

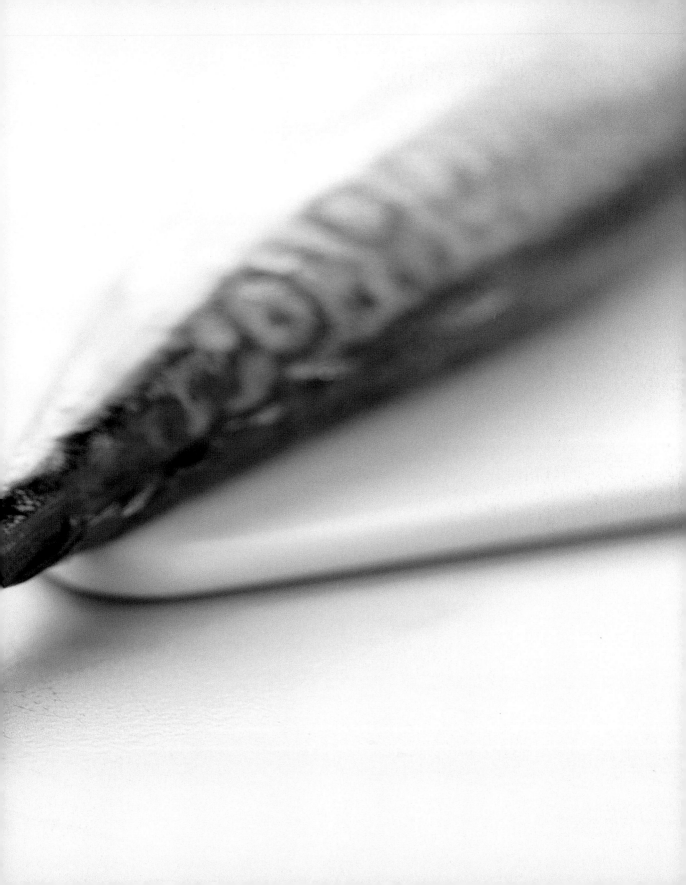

WELL, CONGRATULATIONS. YOU'VE COMPLETED MY 21-DAY HOLISTIC DETOX DIET. YOU SHOULD BE FEELING FULL OF ENERGY, RE-INVIGORATED AND REJUVENATED, WITH A BETTER UNDERSTANDING OF HOW YOUR BODY FUNCTIONS. YOU WILL ALSO BE FEELING MORE ABLE TO COPE WITH THE DAILY CHALLENGES OF WORK, CHILDREN, EMOTIONS AND RELATIONSHIPS.

The maintenance section of the programme is all about how to keep up the good work and hang on to all the benefits you've achieved. Now you have adopted a pattern of eating healthily, and seen the effect it has on your physical, mental and emotional wellbeing, you are in a great position to reintroduce more foods into your diet. Your newly detoxed system will be able to cope – so long as the potentially toxic foods are eaten on an occasional rather than a daily basis. You have cleansed your body so it is now ready to work and perform at an optimum level, so having the odd burger, pizza, chocolate or dessert is not going to do any long-term damage. It may make you feel temporarily sluggish or give you a bit of indigestion but the body will clean itself out again. Do beware, though. If you go out with friends for a pizza, bottle of wine and a tub of ice cream, you may feel quite dreadful afterwards. By restricting yourself to the pizza, say, you give your liver a fighting chance and shouldn't suffer too badly!

It is important that you keep referring to the acid/alkaline chart in Chapter 3. The basis of the maintenance period is the consumption of alkaline foods, particularly fruits and vegetables, which are essential for good digestion and the effective elimination of toxic matter. Continue to shop carefully and to choose nutritious foods. Make sure that you are getting a good supply of amino acids from green leafy vegetables and pulses. In general you should be trying to maintain the quality of everything you're eating, aiming for a low-fat diet and particularly avoiding processed, refined and reduced-fat foods.

The main principle of the maintenance programme is the gradual reintroduction of foods and the careful monitoring of your body's responses. Keep a food diary and note down what you eat and how you feel afterwards. This will enable you to understand how your body reacts to certain foods and to pinpoint any intolerances. For example, you can now start reintroducing sweet fruits such as watermelon, cantaloupe and honeydew melon for breakfast, although it's best to continue to avoid freshly squeezed orange juice since it is so acidic. Instead, try some fresh apricot, banana or melon juice. If you do feel bloated afterwards it is a warning sign that the fruit is fermenting and that you may have an intolerance to fruit and fruit sugers. The important thing from now on is to listen to your body. Be vigilant if it starts to manifest any of those symptoms and problems you experienced BD (Before Detox). If you feel bloated, sluggish or tired or you have indigestion after eating certain foods, try to avoid them in the future.

If dessert is the thing you've been missing, now is the time to reintroduce it. A sorbet is a good choice but ice cream or a slice of cake is not a disaster so long as you have just a small amount. You can start having pasta occasionally (by which I mean about once a week) and even bread if you really want to. Just keep a note of any reactions you experience and adjust your diet accordingly.

Most people, though, actually don't want to revert to their old eating patterns because they find they've got used to the new dietary regime and are enjoying the effect it has on their wellbeing. They feel so much better that they cannot envisage eating the way they did before. The main thing is to keep on track as much as you can. Remember to listen to your body and think of the maintenance programme as the basis of a new way of life rather than a temporary state of affairs.

EATING OUT

Now that you're embarking on the rest of your life and relaxing your restrictions, it's time to plan your new approach to eating out. Because we often see a visit to a restaurant as a treat, we immediately assume that it must be bad for us. And it is – if we opt for cream sauces or shrimp tempura or sticky toffee pudding or cheese for dessert. But look at any menu and any type of cuisine and it is possible to find a healthy option that will fit with the maintenance programme. And remember, because your taste buds will be changing, you won't automatically be drawn to the pasta or French fries you might once have chosen.

Now is the time to experiment with whole sections of the menu that you might not have looked at before. For instance, if you like Thai food, look at the different salads on offer rather than heading straight for the green curries. Similarly, if you normally have the steak in your local French bistro, try looking instead at the fish section where you will probably find some trout or monkfish. The secret is to take control of the menu. Don't feel that you have to eat exactly what is on offer. If the salmon steak comes with a hollandaise sauce ask, instead, for a wedge of lemon. If the chicken is fried ask if it would be possible to grill it instead. And never be afraid of checking what different foods contain and how they are cooked; you are the customer, remember, and your health is at stake. Nowadays many restaurants use well-sourced organic meats and vegetables. And it is a chef's job to be aware of current trends and the fact that many of us are now much more health conscious. So you will nearly always find a 'healthy option' of some sort – even at your local pizza parlour.

One general warning however; it is very easy to eat a couple of bread rolls at the beginning of any meal, almost without thinking about it, because that is when we are most hungry. So in order to stave off any possible temptation, order a bottle of water straight away. A couple of glasses should quell any pangs you might have until your food arrives.

As you begin to discover different parts of the menu so you will find that eating out can be as much a pleasurable part of the maintenance phase of the Holistic Detox as the new foods you have been eating at home. But if you are still nervous of straying off course, here is a guide to set you on your way. Much of this advice focusses on the best possible options and would actually apply as well to the 21-Day Detox as to the maintenance period. Do aim to stick to it, but do also remember that the point of eating out or with friends is to enjoy yourself and that, now you have cleansed your system thoroughly, the odd lapse won't be disastrous.

CHINESE

The most dangerous part of a Chinese menu is the starters section. Please don't go anywhere near the prawn crackers, spring rolls, spare ribs or fried seaweed. Stick, instead, to the chicken satay or a small bowl of chicken and sweetcorn soup. If you would like something a little more indulgent, choose some crispy duck. The pancakes are fine as they are not made from wheat and the spring onion and sliced cucumber accompaniments are perfectly harmless in those quantities. Do make sure to avoid as much of the skin as possible, though, as it is obviously very fattening.

Chicken and vegetable stir fries are a safe option. Beansprouts are packed with nutrients and water chestnuts and Chinese greens are all excellent vitamin-rich choices. Do try to avoid anything in batter and I'm afraid the sweet and sour sauce is also an absolute no-no as it is full of sugar and vinegar. Most Chinese restaurants have an extensive tofu section. As long as the tofu hasn't been fried this is always a good choice although watch out for too many glutinous sauces. You can often tell just by looking at Chinese foods whether they are good for you or not. If a dish looks fresh and clean without too much sauce then it will be fine. Be aware, though, that MSG (a flavour enhancer and artificial stimulant) may be added during cooking. The only way to be sure is to ask.

As with Thai cooking, Chinese menus usually have a very good variety of steamed fish – often with spring onions and ginger. Do, however, go easy on the soy sauce because of the yeast content. If you are passionate about Chinese food it is worth buying some yeast-free soy sauce and taking it out to the restaurant with you. Again, as with Thai food, avoid the fried rice and noodles and choose plain steamed rice instead – sometimes you can find it with saffron, if you feel like something a little more adventurous.

THAI

Thai restaurants offer a wealth of nutritious choices. There is no need to have the prawn toasts or deep-fried spring rolls. Instead, opt for rice paper rolls which are filled with salad, herbs, beansprouts and often a little chicken. And as long as you don't have too much of the peanut sauce, which is very fattening, chicken satay is also another safe choice.

Thai soups are fantastically nourishing as are many of the Thai salads which you can also have as a main course. If you feel the need for something a little more substantial, do try and steer clear of the pork, duck and beef dishes, which are very difficult to digest and full of fat. Instead have chicken, stir fried with ginger and spring onions or with cashew nuts. Minced chicken with basil or ground rice is also a good choice. It's best to avoid very spicy curries as they are very acid-forming. Also avoid the seafood dishes because seafood may contain high levels of mercury and other chemicals. Any other steamed fish – which always features on a Thai menu – would be absolutely fine. It is best not to have noodles as an accompaniment unless they are made of rice. And instead of fried or sticky rice, try to keep to plainly steamed, as it is far less stodgy.

INDIAN

Contrary to what you might expect, it is actually very easy to eat out in an Indian restaurant on the maintenance programme. Choose the paneer – a homemade cottage cheese – as a starter, the sautéed spinach or the grilled chicken tikka.

For a main course it is best to avoid the very hot dishes as too much chilli will cause stomach acid and is bad for the digestion. Also avoid the kormas, which are very mild but too creamy. Instead, head to the house specialities and the tandoori section where you will always find a great selection of grilled tandoori chicken or chicken cooked in a mixture of herbs such as mint, ginger coriander and fenugreek.

Any Indian menu will feature a mixture of different dahls – curried lentils – and often a few chickpea dishes as well. These are excellent choices, full of nutrition and also very low in fat. For accompaniments, pilau rice is a very good option but avoid the nan breads as they are made from wheat flour. Chapatis should be avoided for the same reason. However, it's worth asking if the restaurant has any chapattis made from rye, chick pea, or lentil flour. Popadoms are fine as they are made from rice but ask for them to be grilled rather than deep fried. As a dip choose the raita, which is made from yoghurt and mint, rather than the chutney which is high in sugar.

ITALIAN

Italian cuisine can be a bit trickier. Buffalo mozzarella is a good choice to start with, in a salad with tomatoes. Most restaurants will also offer avocado which is fine as long as you have only a little vinaigrette.

Try to avoid choosing the pasta dishes or pizzas as your standard option. Risottos are a better choice, especially if you're vegetarian. Or look instead to the meat and fish section where you will always find a simple grilled chicken, fish or veal dish. Roast partridge is also fine. Instead of the different sauces, which are often full of oil and butter, ask for a wedge of lemon. A good Italian restaurant will have a varied choice of vegetable side orders. Try the cavalo nero (black cabbage), the spinach or the fresh broad beans. Sometimes these will be served with feta cheese, which is fine in small quantities as it is made from sheep's milk. If you see this on the side orders menu it also makes a good starter – don't be afraid to mix and match.

The chain pizza restaurants now offer a wide range of salads. Choose a chicken based salad or the tuna nicoise. Treat the Caesar salads as an occasional treat as the dressing is exceptionally high in fat and it is difficult to digest the Parmesan cheese.

Funnily enough, breadsticks are all right as they have no yeast, but they do contain small amounts of wheat, so until you are confident about your body's response to wheat, you should eat them sparingly.

JAPANESE

Japanese cuisine is generally one of the cleanest and healthiest in the world, making it a very easy choice, even on the 21-Day Detox and certainly in the maintenance phase.

Order a bowl of *edamame* – soya beans – to pick at while you decide what to choose. There's always a brilliant range of salads, often with chargrilled salmon, tuna or chicken. Most restaurants also do a spinach dish topped with toasted sesame seeds and spring onion. *Yakitori* – chargrilled chicken skewers – are another excellent choice for a starter. The only thing you really need to avoid are the *tempura*, which means anything that's deep fried in batter, and the *gyoza* which are little dumplings made of flour and filled with prawns, chicken or vegetables.

I recommend *sushi* and *sashimi*, which are always satisfying, virtually fat free, and surprisingly filling. Another good choice would be the *ramen* (noodle soups) with bean sprouts and herbs. Choose the salmon or chicken *ramen* and ask for rice noodles rather than egg. *Miso* soups are also incredibly nutritious and often come with vegetables, chicken or tofu. Do remember, though, that they contain yeast, and so may make you feel bloated.

Any of the chicken, fish or vegetable noodle dishes are also good but again, ask for rice noodles rather than egg. *Bento* boxes – or Japanese lunch boxes – consist of an assortment of chicken, fish and vegetables and come with pickles, steamed rice and salad. (Do eat the pickles sparingly, though, as they contain vinegar.) The only other thing you should really try to avoid in a Japanese restaurant is the *don buri* – vegetables or meat coated in breadcrumbs and then deep fried.

FRENCH

French restaurants are fine as long as you avoid regular splurges on the classic French sauces such as hollandaise and béarnaise which are basically a hot mayonnaise and therefore high in oil and vinegar.

Soup is often the best choice of starter, particularly if there is a fresh vegetable soup of the day. You will also normally find a good selection of fish such as salt cod, anchovies or smoked salmon.

Instead of choosing the steaks, which are such a staple of the French cuisine, look instead at the chicken and fish sections. There will always be at least three or four choices, which you can ask to be plainly grilled rather than smothered in sauce. As with Italians, a French restaurant always has a good choice of vegetable side orders. So instead of frites, ask for green beans, fresh peas or whatever that day's selection of green vegetables happens to be.

RALPH'S STORY

I've been receiving treatment from Nish Joshi for four years. He was recommended to me by the Almeida theatre while I was working there in 2000. I pretty much regard him as my GP as he has helped me with a variety of conditions that an orthodox medic could not, and he would be the first person I'd turn to for medical advice.

He has used acupuncture on me to heal a strained shoulder muscle that was being over-stressed in a stage fight, and he sent me a medicinal drink, for a bad bronchial infection I was suffering, while I was performing Coriolanus in Tokyo. He didn't hesitate to send the bottle out to me and it cleared up the infection within forty-eight hours. You wouldn't find too many GPs who would do that! I also find him to be an extremely positive character.

I am not a vegetarian, and I do drink coffee and alcohol, but I do listen to his advice on diet even though I don't follow it to extremes.

RALPH FIENNES, 41, STAR OF THE FILM *THE ENGLISH PATIENT*, WAS INTRODUCED TO JOSHI WHILE PERFORMING AT A LONDON THEATRE. SINCE THEN, HE AND FRANCESCA ANNIS, HIS ACTRESS PARTNER, HAVE TRUSTED HIM WITH THEIR MEDICAL CARE.

MIDDLE EASTERN

The beauty of Middle Eastern restaurants is that they usually involve mezze – a series of small individual dishes which are easy to mix and match.

Choose the hummus, *tzatsiki*, or *baba ghanoush*, a pureed aubergine dish. Along with pitta bread, ask for some chopped carrots to dip. Falafels which are made from ground up chick peas and spices are another good choice. Avoid the couscous and tabbouleh which both contain wheat, instead choose a chicken *kibbeh* which is a ground meat patty, or maybe grilled chicken with a lemon and garlic sauce. Don't touch the fried pastries filled with cheese or minced meat but do have the grilled quail with cinnamon and the delicious, delicately spiced, salads.

AMERICAN DINERS

Believe it or not, you can even eat out at one of the American style chain restaurants. Obviously the choice will be a bit limited as I do urge you to continue to refuse the burger or hot dog and chips, or at least to regard them as a very occasional treat, but with a little imagination and some help from the kitchen it is possible to have a healthy, enjoyable meal.

Soup is, as always, a very good choice for a starter. As a main course, focus on salads or order a chicken club sandwich and ask the kitchen to turn it into salad, without the bread. There's also usually a salad nicoise or a house salad to choose from, but please avoid saturating it in Thousand Island dressing. Nowadays diner restaurants even offer a fish option – usually a chargrilled salmon fillet served with vegetables or a salad.

DETOX FOR LIFE

Now you have your diet sorted you may be ready to focus on the broader aspects of detox. This is time to exploit the great new you – and your feelings of invigoration, energy, and new-found confidence in your slimmer, trimmer figure. Hopefully, by now you should like yourself a lot more, feel more attractive and value yourself more highly, all of which puts you in the prefect place to re-evaluate your relationships, work patterns and home environment in order to keep introducing positive changes to your life. There are two things, in addition to a good diet, from which I find people gain particular support as they adapt their lives during the maintenance period: physical exercise and, especially, Ayurvedic practice.

The benefits of regular physical exercise are well-known and are absolutely crucial to the maintenance of a healthy body and mind. Try to use this time to increase your level of exercise if you can, particularly if you would like to shed a few more pounds. Even if you are not aiming for further significant weight loss, aerobic and weight-bearing exercise is vital during the maintenance period in order to encourage the body to use its fat stores rather than looking to muscle for its energy. Exercising decreases the chance that your body will adjust to its new calorie intake and over-compensate, creating a yo-yo dieting effect. If you reduce the amount of calories you ingest but do not increase your exercise rate, your metabolic rate is likely to start to slow down. This can lead to weight re-gain.

On my Holistic Detox you're helping the body to break down fat cells by getting more active and taking more exercise. Simultaneously, you're encouraging the liver to detoxify so that it eliminates toxins, stimulants and chemicals rather than storing them in fat. This double-whammy results in a leaner, healthier more energised body and mind.

One other thing to reiterate about the maintenance phase of the programme: keep up your fluid intake, especially if you're exercising more. A constant flow of filtered water is essential to your liver functioning and to the avoidance of dehydration. Remember, getting fit is thirsty work!

THE AYURVEDIC WAY

Ayurveda, the traditional holistic medicine of India, offers one of the most effective ways to improve our health, increase our energy, focus our mind, and shift those stubborn excess pounds. The fundamental aim of Ayurveda – and the Joshi Holistic Detox Programme – is to encourage you to take control of your wellbeing, both physical and spiritual, by achieving a better balance between your body and your mind.

For thousands of years in India and the East medical disciplines have relied upon re-establishing harmony within the body as a means of restoring good health and treating illness. Physicians do not separate out the physical from the mental or emotional wellbeing of the patient, which are considered to be parts of the whole and treated concurrently. In the West, this concept of holistic health care is still somewhat alien in that doctors tend to treat the physical symptoms of an illness rather than its cause, and rarely consider other aspects of the patient's life such as his mental or emotional wellbeing.

As an Indian Brahmin I was brought up to follow the teachings of Ayurveda, which is not just a medicine or a treatment but an entire way of life that seeks to balance the body using a combination of diet, exercise, meditation and herbal supplements. The results of making Ayurvedic balance central to your on-going maintenance programme will be miraculous. Not only will you feel increasingly energised, you will also literally glow, inside and out, and you may even find that you have no further need of your painkillers, blood pressure pills and cholesterol tablets.

At the heart of Ayurveda is the creation of harmony. But we can only achieve this if we have a complete picture of who we are. One of the easiest ways to understand this is to imagine the mind, soul and body as a tripod and the need for all three to be balanced to ensure that whatever it is supporting doesn't fall down.

Because we are all individual, of different shapes and sizes, with varied metabolisms, living in different environments, some of us single living alone, some married with children, some stressed, some relaxed, some working, some caring, our digestive processes and reactions to food will be different. The Ayurvedic route, however, is founded on the knowledge that each person is different. It is therefore the perfect tool to help you tweak your diet during the maintenance phase in order to maximise the benefits of the 21-Day Detox.

Normally, an Ayurvedic physician would not only make a thorough physical examination of a patient to find out any pathological conditions but also gain a knowledge of his or her mental state and enduring traits. He must know the patient's social background and the geographical and cultural context in which they live. With a basic understanding of the Ayurvedic doctrine we can establish these factors ourselves and so achieve maximum benefit from the on-going Detox programme.

Ayurvedic philosophy is based on the fact that everything in this universe is made up of the five great elements or building blocks – earth, water, fire, air and ether. Although matter is a mixture of these five elements there is usually one element that's predominant. So, for example, a mountain is mainly made up of earth but also contains water, fire, air and ether.

UNDERSTANDING DOSHAS

Ayurveda teaches that this law of nature also applies to our selves. Hence it divides the human body into one of three metabolic types, or *doshas*, which are based on different pairings of these elements. So:

⇢ Air and ether combine to form the *Vata dosha*
⇢ Water and earth combine to form the *Kapha dosha*
⇢ Fire and water combine to form the *Pitta dosha*

According to Ayurvedic principle our health and wellbeing are fundamentally dependent on the balance of these three *doshas*. To begin with, these terms might sound strange. But when you realise how it works, Ayurveda makes perfect sense. By completing the chart on page 120 you can establish which *dosha* is most prominent in you. And then I promise you a fascinating journey on which you will discover your strengths and weaknesses and find out how to reshape and support your body by altering your diet in relation to the balance of the three *doshas*. The chart on page 128 will explain which food groups particularly affect each *dosha* and how to create balance.

All three *doshas* are present through the body but each one is predominant in different places and therefore they perform different, specific, functions.

Vata

In line with the nature of its elements, air and ether, *Vata* governs motion and movement. It is responsible for breathing, the swallowing of food, the circulation of the blood and the health of the heart. It is also involved with the flow of nerve impulses to and from the brain, controls the flow of liquids in the body and helps in the action of the digestive enzymes. *Vata* controls the urinary system and the reproductive organs. Its function is to hold the faeces, urine and semen up to a normal period and then expel them through the various channels of the body.

When *Vata* is out of balance, symptoms can include distension of the gut, bloating, constipation, fatigue, stiff and painful joints, heart palpitations and fainting spells.

Kapha

Kapha, like its elements, earth and water, is solid and steady by nature and is the heaviest of the three *doshas*. *Kapha* provides the body's structure and lubrication. It controls fluid balance and governs the production of phlegm and mucus. It also moistens the food in the stomach by creating humidity within the body and is responsible for lubrication of joints, so preventing any excessive friction from occurring. This also helps prevent arthritic changes. *Kapha* is the *dosha* that gives us strength by forming muscle, fat, bone and sinew. It also plays a huge role in increasing appetite.

Signs of a *Kapha* imbalance include nausea, aching joints, heavy limbs and congestion in the nose or sinuses. Imbalance can also lead to lethargy and weight gain.

Pitta

Consistent with its two main elements, fire and water, *Pitta* is the main driver of the body. It governs metabolism and the digestion of food, breaking down the matter into essential enzymes and dividing out that which is useful and that which is waste. *Pitta* maintains the body's temperature, helps in memory function and intellect, and controls our vision, converting external images into optic nerve impulses. It is also the *dosha* that influences our complexion, giving colour and softness to the skin.

A *Pitta* imbalance can lead to fitful sleep, diarrhoea, hot flushes, skin rashes and acne, fevers and sweats and bloodshot eyes.

YOUR AYURVEDIC METABOLIC TYPE

Just as in nature, the three *doshas* occur in everyone; but while all three of them are active, the proportion varies according to the individual and one or two usually dominate. It is because we are all born with our own unique combination of the three *doshas* that people can have much in common but also an endless variety of differences in the way they behave and respond to their environment, including their diet.

This unique combination is known as your Ayurvedic metabolic type. The self-diagnosis chart on page 120 will help you identify which main *dosha* you correspond to and where your imbalances are. Once you have established this, the aim is to keep the three *doshas* and the relationship between them in balance. I should stress that this is something you should pay constant attention to as within each person the *doshas* are continually interacting with one another and with the *doshas* in all of nature. This is not as difficult as it might at first sound. Once you have learnt to understand your body and the warning signs it will give you when there is an imbalance, adjusting your diet and lifestyle accordingly will become second nature.

And when you have achieved balance between the three *doshas* you will experience health on all levels: mental, physical and spiritual. This is what makes Ayurveda so special: it maximises the body's full potential, taking it to new heights of wellbeing. It is about so much more than the mere prevention and absence of disease.

Conversely, when the *doshas* are unbalanced – when one or more of the *dosha* levels has either increased or decreased – then we become susceptible to sickness and a myriad physical disorders. Uncovering the fundamental cause of any ailment, according to Ayurvedic principles, is achieved by identifying the main *dosha* that has been imbalanced, be it *Kapha*, *Vata* or *Pitta*.

Even if we are not experienced Ayurvedic physicians we can learn a lot about our health from an Ayurvedic perspective, through self-diagnosis, either by taking our temperature or pulse-rate, or examining our tongue. If, for example, we have indentations on the side of our tongue, it may indicate that we have a *Pitta* imbalance, while a thick coating would signal a *Vata* imbalance. There are guidelines on tongue analysis on page 87.

Of course I do not suggest that you use an Ayurvedic diagnosis instead of visiting your GP. If you feel you have a medical problem or symptoms of a condition that warrants attention, do not hesitate to visit your doctor. And I should stress that Ayurveda does not deny the existence of bacteria or viruses or their role in creating disease in the body, but it does give more importance to the nature of the person being affected by it. Some people, as we know, are by nature more susceptible to colds, some to windy troubles and some to bilious problems. No Ayurvedic physician can prescribe the same medication to each person, even if they have fallen sick with the same disease. That is why Ayurvedic diagnosis appears more subjective than conventional Western diagnosis: because it treats the person as a whole rather than simply treating the condition.

USING THE AYURVEDIC CHART

I would like you to complete the self-diagnosis chart, which will enable you to determine your unique constitution according to Ayurvedic principles. But please remember that this can only provide a rough guide, not a cast-iron definition, as the subtleties of each person's mental, emotional and physical make up are manifold and can be accurately assessed only by a physician thoroughly trained and experienced in Ayurvedic diagnosis. You can, however, use the information you gather to help you plan your diet, exercise regime and other aspects of your lifestyle for maximum health and use it on a weekly basis to monitor improvements. It is best therefore to revisit the chart at the beginning of each week you choose to continue the maintenance. You will notice each time you check the list how your *doshas* change, how the balance shifts, and how you can affect and harmonise your health, moving towards equilibrium. You may well instinctively understand what you need to do in order to balance your profile, but the chart is invaluable for pinpointing the severity of your symptoms and planning effective long term reconditioning. It's a great way to encourage you to keep on track, too.

It is often useful for a friend or partner to take a look at your answers, as they may be more objective than you can be about your responses. For each category, such as skin type or body type, make a note of whether you most resemble *vata*, *kapha* or *pitta* characteristics. Then total up your scores to discover which *dosha* you lean towards and where your imbalances are.
Most people will have one *dosha* prominent, a few will have two *doshas* approximately equal and even fewer will have all three *doshas* in equal proportion. In order to get the clearest sense of the relative proportions of your *doshas*, you can,

after adding up the numbers, divide each column total by three to make three the highest number; i.e. if your score for *Vata* was ten, *Pitta* six and *Kapha* three, this would translate into a score of *Vata* three, *Pitta* two and *Kapha* one. Since *Kapha* is the dominant *dosha*, if you have a perfectly even score you should read the advice for those with a high *Kapha* score and implement some of the suggestions. Since you don't have an imbalance, though, you need only tweak, rather than overhaul your diet and lifestyle.

Once you have determined your predominant *dosha*, study the guidelines to the typical characteristics of *Vata*, *Pitta* and *Kapha*. Once you have an understanding of your metabolic type you can move on to consider how to balance it more effectively by using the Ayurvedic food charts on pages 127 and 128 to adapt your diet and lifestyle.

AYURVEDIC METABOLIC TYPE CHART

CHARACTERISTIC	VATA	KAPHA	PITTA	YOUR METABOLIC TYPE (V, K OR P)
Body weight	Low	Overweight	Average	P
Body Size	Slim	Large	Average	V
Skin Type	Thin, dry, rough, dark, cold	Thick, oily, cool, white, pale,	Smooth, oily, warm, rosy	K (P) V
Nails	Dry, rough, brittle, thin	Thick, oily, smooth, polished	Sharp, flexible, luminescent, pink	V
Eyes	Small, sunken, animated	Big, calm, soft	Sharp, bright, sensitive to light	P
Hair	Dry, brown/black, brittle, thin	Thick, wavy/curly, oily, lustrous	Straight, oily, blonde/grey/red, bald	V
Lips	Dry, cracked, black/brown, tinged	Smooth, oily, pale, white	Red, inflamed	K P
Chin	Thin, angular	Rounded, double	Tapering	K P
Cheeks	Wrinkled, sunken	Rounded, plump	Smooth, flat	P
Neck	Thin, taught, long	Big, folded	Smooth, flat	P
Chest	Flat, sunken	Rounded, pendulous	Average	P
Belly	Flat, sunken	Rounded, extended	Average	V
Hips	Slender, thin	Heavy, rounded	Average	V
Joints	Cold, crack a lot	Large, move freely	Average	P
Digestion	Irregular, gassy	Slow, forming soft stools	Quick, burning sensation, acidic	V
Appetite	Irregular, scant	Slow, steady	Strong, always hungry, eating often	K
Cravings	Sweet, sour, salty	Bitter, pungent, astringent	Sweet, bitter, astringent	V
Thirst	Changeable	Sparse	Surplus	P
Elimination	Constipated	Thick/sluggish	Loose	K
Physical activity	Hyper	Sedentary	Moderate	V
Mental activity	Hyper	Slow thinking	Moderate	V
Emotions	Anxious, fearful, nervy	Calm, needy	Extreme swings	K
Intellect	Quick, spontaneous	Slow, exact	Precise	V P
Memory	Short term good, long term poor	Slow and sustained	Distinct, clear	P
Dreams	Quick, active, prone to nightmares	Romantic, pleasant, calm	Fiery and violent	V
Sleep	Insomniac, broken	Deep, long, uninterrupted	Little but sound	P
Speech	Rapid, unclear	Slow, monotone	Sharp, distinct	P

Vata total: 9 /3

Kapha total: 5

Pitta total: 13

Dominant dosha: P

UNDERSTANDING YOUR DOSHA TYPE

Vata ✓

The word *Vata* is derived from the Sanskrit word meaning 'to move' and this gives an important clue to the character of a *Vata* individual. *Vatas* tend to have light, flexible bodies. Their frames tend to be on the small side, with light muscles and little fat because they can't stop moving and fidgeting. They are usually slim or even under-weight. They often appear to be too tall or too short and may be physically under-developed with flat chests and less strength and stamina than the other types. Their veins and muscles are often quite prominent.

APPETITE These individuals have a variable appetite and thirst and variable digestive strength. They often crave astringent foods like salads and vegetables but because their digestion can be poor, *Vatas* should be wary of eating these in large quantities. They tend to produce scanty urine, their faeces are hard and dry, small in size and quantity, and constipation is one of their biggest problems.

CIRCULATION *Vatas* generally have dry skin, tending even towards roughness. Their circulation is poor with the result that their hands and feet are often cold. Because the *Vata dosha* is cold and dry, light and mobile, people with a *Vata* constitution tend to lack insulating material, i.e. the fatty tissue under the skin. They are uncomfortable in cold weather, especially if it is dry and windy and they much prefer spring and summer.

PHYSICAL TRAITS *Vatas* are the most likely of the body types to fast or eat very little. But this actually increases the *Vata dosha* and therefore produces a tendency towards imbalance. Other physical characteristics typical of *Vata* types include: small, deep-set sunken eyes which lack lustre; dry, thin hair, often curly or kinky; dry, rough skin and nails. Their joints tend to crack a lot and their teeth may be irregular or protruding.

MOVEMENT AND SEX *Vata* types tend to move quite quickly as it is the *dosha* of movement and they are always in a rush. They do not like sitting idle, but prefer constant activity and they also like to travel. *Vatas* are also drawn towards a lot of sexual activity but excess sex is one of the causes of an aggravated *Vata*! *Vatas* generally have a difficult time prolonging sex and *Vata* men may experience premature ejaculation.

MENTAL AGILITY *Vata* individuals sleep less than other types and have a tendency towards either interrupted sleep or insomnia, especially when *Vata* is aggravated. Nevertheless, they do tend to wake up feeling alert and fresh and ready to go again. Psychologically, *Vatas* are blessed with quick minds, mental flexibility, and creativity. They have excellent imaginations and excel in coming up with lots of ideas. When in balance they are joyful and happy people, who tend to talk a lot. They are excited quickly and are alert and quick to act and react. However, they do not always think things through and as a result they tend to make wrong decisions and often suffer from poor self-confidence.

FEARS AND WORRIES *Vatas* are loving people but may love out of fear and loneliness. In fact, fear is one of the symptoms of an imbalanced *Vata dosha*. *Vata* individuals may experience fear of loneliness, darkness, heights and closed spaces. Anxiety, insecurity and nervousness are also common fears. *Vatas* are the worriers.

CHANGE AND FLEXIBILITY One of the main psychological qualities of *Vata* individuals is their readiness to change. Or, to put it in another way, they have a difficulty with stability and commitment so they often move on from people, jobs, houses and towns. They get bored easily and they are quite low on will power.

IMPULSIVE AND CLEARSIGHTED Clarity is one of the attributes of *Vata* individuals who are clear-minded and can even be clairvoyant. With their lively minds and fertile imaginations, they grasp new ideas quickly. However, they are also quick to forget and they think and speak quickly but are restless and easily fatigued. They generally have less tolerance, confidence, and boldness than other types. *Vata* types make money quickly but they also spend it quickly and are quite impulsive in their nature.

IMBALANCES *Vatas* fidget and can't sit still for long periods of time, which is why they are drawn to travel, erratic hours, continual stimulation and frequent change. The trouble is that this can easily upset their balance and lead to disorders such as arthritis, pneumonia, excessively dry skin, dry lips, dry hair, dry cracked nipples and cracked heels, nervous disorders, mental confusion, muscle tightness, back pain and sciatica. *Vata* types can also suffer from restlessness and hyperactivity. Loud noises, drugs, sugar, caffeine, alcohol can also cause imbalance as can exposure to cold weather and cold foods.

Excess *Vata* is a major factor in pre-menstrual syndrome (PMS) and produces such symptoms as bloating, lower back pain, pain in the lower abdomen, cramps, pain in the calf, insomnia and emotional anxiety. Insecurity is another indication of an aggravated Vata dosha as is an excess of wind.

Sticking to a routine is difficult for *Vata* types but it is vital if they are to remain healthy. A general piece of advice on balancing an excess of *Vata* is to keep warm and calm and avoid raw and cold foods. Instead eat warm foods and spices and maintain a regular routine.

Pitta

The *Pitta* type is usually of medium height and build, although some have a slender or delicate frame. *Pittas* tend to be stronger than *Vatas*, and have coppery skin and reddish silky hair. Moles and freckles are common on *Pitta* skin, which tends to be oily, warm and less wrinkled than a *Vata* complexion. *Pittas* have sharp, yellowish teeth and can occasionally complain of bleeding gums. They also tend to have a higher metabolic temperature, and a higher metabolic rate than other individuals.

APPETITE *Pittas* have a strong appetite, strong metabolism and a strong digestion. They consume large quantities of food and drink, and they also produce large quantities of urine and faeces, which tends to be usually yellowish and soft. When out of balance they love to eat hot spicy dishes, which are not good for them. They should eat food with sweet, bitter and astringent tastes. When hungry, a *Pitta* person needs to eat immediately otherwise he or she will become irritable or hypoglycaemic.

HEAT AND SEX *Pittas* perspire a lot even when other people around them are freezing. An excess of heat is the main characteristic of the Pitta individual and in fact the word *Pitta* is Sanskrit for heat. *Pitta* people also tend to be fiery in their personality. Curiously, their sex drive is not that strong but they tend to use sex as a means to release anger.

FIERY AILMENTS *Pitta* sleep is usually of medium duration but it is uninterrupted and quite sound.

They like to read before they nod off and often fall asleep with the TV on or with a book on their chest. *Pitta* people tend to suffer from physical ailments related to heat and the fire principle, and are prone to fevers, inflammatory diseases, acidic indigestion, excessive hunger, jaundice, lots of perspiration, rashes, ulceration, burning eyes, colitis, sore throats as well as being particularly susceptible to sunburn and heartburn. *Pitta* women tend to menstruate from a young age and suffer PMS symptoms. These include tenderness of the breasts, hot flushes and hives. They are vulnerable to cystitis.

INTELLECT *Pitta* types tend to be alert and intelligent and have good powers of comprehension and concentration. Their intellects are keen and penetrating and their memories sharp. They also have good logical and investigative minds which are always alert and constantly at work. They love to delve deeply into problems and find their solutions. *Pittas* also tend to be good speakers. They enjoy learning and have a great capacity for organisation and leadership.

ORDERLY NIGHT OWLS *Pittas* tend to be night people and are often at their most alert around midnight. If there is no one to play with they will read into the small hours. Orderliness is also important to them. A *Pitta's* home is always clean and neat. Clothes are kept in a designated place, shoes are in orderly rows, and books are arranged according to height or other defining systems. *Pittas* tend to love the professions so many are doctors, engineers, lawyers, or judges.

IMBALANCES *Pitta* imbalances can be increased by sour and citrus fruits such as grapefruit and oranges, and by rancid yoghurt, smoking cigarettes, and drinking sour wine. Working near fire and lying in the sun can cause an excess

imbalance too. Eating fatty fried foods or oily foods, such as peanut butter, can cause nausea or headaches for a *Pitta* individual.

Summer is the most difficult time for *Pitta* people. They become particularly aggravated during hot humid weather. Heat builds up in the system so the *Pitta* individuals become more susceptible to the heat-related ailments mentioned above. They may become irritable and easily agitated and angered. That's when tempers can flare. They tend to have hypercritical, judgemental minds. Jealousy and envy are common traits and more often than not *Pittas* just need to cool down.

Guidelines for balancing *Pitta* include: avoiding excessive heat, oil, steam, and salt. Eating cooling non-spicy foods, drinking cool but not iced drinks, and exercising during the cooler part of the day, will keep *Pittas* on track.

Kapha

Kapha people are blessed with strong, healthy, well-developed bodies.

Their chests are broad and expansive and they have strong muscles and large heavy bones. With their larger frames and their constitutions dominated by the water and earth elements *Kaphas* tend, however, to be prone to weight gain and have difficulty losing weight. To complicate matters, *Kaphas* generally have a slow digestion and metabolism. In addition to their large frames, *Kapha* individuals have strong stamina and tend to be very healthy. Their skin is usually soft and oily. Their eyes are large, dark and attractive and they have long, thick lashes and brows. The whites of their eyes are often bright white and they have strong, large white teeth.

Kaphas tend to be sluggish with their digestion so they evacuate their faeces slowly and their stools tend to be soft and pale in colour. They perspire more than *Vatas* and less than *Pittas*. Their sleep is usually deep and prolonged, but they wake up feeling more sluggish than refreshed. Because of the heavy qualities of *Kapha*, these individuals often feel heavy and foggy in the morning and may find it hard to get moving without a cup of coffee or tea. Morning is not their time, they prefer midday but might feel like taking a nap after lunch. They often feel lethargic after a full meal and unfortunately daytime naps are not good for them.

APPETITE Individuals with *Kapha* body types have a steady appetite and thirst. Their digestion is slow, so they can comfortably skip a meal or work without food. Because of their slow metabolic rate *Kaphas* who maintain health and balance generally enjoy a longer life span than the other two *dosha* types who burn out more quickly. However, if the *Kapha dosha* is allowed to become aggravated, the individual will be vulnerable to obesity, which is one of the main causes of diabetes, hypertension and heart attack.

Kaphas have quite a sweet tooth and love cakes, chocolates and biscuits. They are generally attracted to sweet, salty and oily foods but these contribute to water retention and weight gain. They need to reduce the intake of these foods and instead opt for bitter, astringent and pungent tastes.

WATERY AILMENTS Physical problems with *Kapha* individuals tend to be water-related, such as colds, 'flu, sinusitis and other diseases involving mucus, such as bronchial congestion, sluggishness, excessive weight gain, diabetes, water retention, and headaches.

EXERCISE Despite their strong bodies and great stamina *Kaphas* shun exercise. Vigorous exercise is good for them, but they prefer to walk slowly rather than jog, for example. They do like swimming but it is not particularly good for them as their bodies absorb water they don't need. When they do exercise they become hungry afterwards so after a work out at the gym, they will go straight for a snack, often of cakes and biscuits.

MENTAL AND EMOTIONAL QUALITIES *Kapha dosha* is slow and steady in every way. *Kapha* individuals move slowly and gracefully, talk slowly, eat slowly and are slow to decide and slow to act. They are blessed with a sweet loving disposition. By nature they are peaceful, patient, caring, compassionate, tolerant and forgiving people who make excellent friends as they are faithful and steady. One of the dominant qualities of a *Kapha* individual is the softness they manifest: of skin and hair as well as speech and demeanour.

Kaphas are quite slow to comprehend, but once they know something their knowledge is permanently retained and they have excellent long-term memories. Beware upsetting a *Kapha* type – they may forgive, but are unlikely to forget.

STEADY LOVERS A *Kapha* person has a steady sex drive and can enjoy sex for hours at a time without dissipation of energy, without orgasm and even without ejaculation. It can take some time for them to become interested but once they are stimulated they tend to stay that way.

IMBALANCES A *Kapha dosha* is aggravated by *Kapha*-producing food such as watermelon and other sweet fruits, sweets, biscuits, yoghurt, dairy produce, cold and frozen food and chilled water. Sleeping in the daytime and sitting doing nothing all day will also create a *Kapha* imbalance, as will sedentary work, especially when combined with steady munching at a desk. An excess of *Kapha* slows digestion and metabolism and lowers the digestive fire, or the *Pitta*, that *Kapha* types need. In these circumstances a *Kapha* person may become overweight or even obese.

Winter and early spring are difficult times for *Kapha* individuals since when the weather is heavy, wet and cold the *Kapha,* or mucous, that accumulates in the system leads to physical, emotional and mental imbalances. Emotionally, when a *Kapha* person becomes unbalanced he or she can suffer from greed, envy, possessiveness, lust and laziness leading to a *Kapha*-type depression. Interestingly, *Kapha* can become aggravated as the moon waxes because biologists have discovered that there is a tendency towards water retention in the body at that time.

Since water is the defining quality of a *Kapha* individual, *Kapha* women may suffer from PMS symptoms such as exaggerated emotions, water retention, a white vaginal discharge, over urination.

A basic guideline for balancing *Kapha* is to keep active, maintain a varied routine, get plenty of exercise, and avoid heavy foods, particularly mucous-producing dairy products, iced foods and anything oily or fatty. Instead eat light, dry foods.

BALANCING YOUR DOSHAS

In a nutshell, a *Kapha* individual is rather like a cuddly bear, while a *Vata* type is more like a Siamese cat, very sinewy and graceful. Meanwhile, a *Pitta* person most resembles a Jack Russell terrier, running around all over the place. The ideal is to introduce elements of a counter-balancing *dosha,* so, for example, the *Kapha* person who is a bit sluggish needs some *Pitta* to perk him up, which he can attain by eating some *Pitta*-aggravating spicy foods. He would also benefit from more exercise to get him moving faster and some time in a colder climate – a skiing trip would be ideal!

Conversely, the *Pitta* type needs to relax more and practise some meditation exercises, or take up yoga rather than over-stimulate the body in the gym. *Pitta* people need to avoid foods that are going to irritate or aggravate them such as caffeine, alcohol, and spicy foods.

The *Vata* person tends to have a lot of natural nervous energy so he needs to do some gentle exercise like Pilates or yoga and must ensure he gets adequate sleep, perhaps by listening to relaxation tapes or drinking camomile tea. It's a good idea to avoid too many raw vegetables too, since they increase rather than balance *vata*.

High Vata Score

High *Vata* scorers should avoid all astringent, pungent and bitter foods, as these will only accentuate their more hyperactive symptoms, as will stimulants such as caffeine and chocolate. *Vata* types need to calm down so you should go for sweet, sour and salty foods and eat them slowly. Hot dishes are better than cold and cooked food is preferable to raw. Gentle meditation and relaxing yoga exercises are a better idea than high impact physical activity. Adopting elements of a *Kapha*-promoting diet will keep hyper *Vatas* in balance.

High Kapha score

If you have a high *Kapha* score, you need to eat more pungent foods (onions, radishes, garlic, ginger, cumin), bitter foods (green leafy vegetables such as spinach, bitter greens, turmeric) and astringent foods (lentils, broccoli, cabbage) to help stimulate digestion. Combine these foods with more raw vegetables, salads and lots of fibre to really give your sluggish digestive system a boost. Even a small amount of tea or coffee (just one cup a day) is useful to speed things up a little – all things in moderation. High-scoring *Kaphas* must be particularly careful not to give in to sweet or salty snacks since these things will make them feel more lethargic and bloated as well as heavier. They also need to increase their *Pitta dosha,* by eating spicier foods and taking more exercise. Time to get the bear out of the chair and start mimicking that Jack Russell.

High Pitta score

Men in particular, who are trying to maintain muscle bulk or who lose weight quickly, frequently find that they have a high *Pitta* score. If your *Pitta* is quite high then your *Vata* will be too and your *Kapha* will be correspondingly low. You need to increase your intake of foods that will suppress your heightened stimulation. You should stay away from salty foods, spicy foods, cold and fizzy drinks. Your goal is to increase your *Kapha* score so you should opt for energy-rich foods such as potatoes, meat and eggs. To limit your *Vata* imbalance you should also concentrate on meditation exercises (see page 150 for a simple technique) to help your mind calm down, and some gentle yoga to optimise breathing techniques. Try to work these exercises into your daily routine in order to see accelerated rates of improvement in your symptoms.

AYURVEDIC FOOD GROUPS

Ayurveda divides food into six tastes: sour, salty, sweet, astringent, bitter and pungent. There's a brief guide to these taste groups opposite and also a *dosha*-specific food chart which details balancing foods for each metabolic type. You will see that I have included foods that are not allowed on the 21-Day Detox; but now you are moving into the maintenance phase of my Holistic Detox Programme, and are re-introducing foods to your diet, it's vital to have a good understanding of their impact on your Ayurvedic profile.

SIX TASTES CHART

SOUR
Foods: Yogurt, vinegar, cheese, sour cream, green grapes, lemon (and other citrus fruits), tamarind, pickles, and herbs such as coriander, and cloves.
Effect: Reduces Vata, increases Pitta, increases Kapha. Stimulates appetite and sharpens the mind. Although foods are acidic they will slow the metabolism.

SALTY
Foods: Table salt, sea salt, rock salt, crisps, marine fish, vegetables; remember, there is also a lot of salt in tinned and processed foods, which should always be avoided where possible.
Effect: Reduces Vata, increases Pitta, increases Kapha. Helps digestion; acts as a laxative.

SWEET
Foods: Fruits, sugar, cakes, honey, syrup, molasses, certain vegetables such as carrots and beets, dairy produce, rice, bread. I recommend that you continue to avoid highly processed sweets such as candy bars and sugar.
Effect: Reduces Vata, reduces Pitta, increases Kapha. Excessive amounts of sugar will make you put on weight. The problem with eating sugary foods such as chocolate and cakes is that they also contain additives, food colourants and preservatives, which will have an adverse affect on your fat levels. Fizzy drinks can also raise your Vata.

ASTRINGENT
Foods: Vinegar, pickles, unripe banana, cranberries, pomegranate.
Effect: Increases Vata, reduces Pitta, reduces Kapha. Astringent foods can promote healing as they have a sedative action but they also produce a lot of gas and acid.

PUNGENT
Foods: Onion, pickles, spices, aromatic foods, chilli, ginger, garlic, mustard.
Effect: Increases Vata, increases Pitta, reduces Kapha. Spices stimulate digestive juices and increase production of acid, which will raise your Pitta. Also helps with Kapha problem of obesity, slow digestion.

BITTER
Foods: Coffee, wine, alcohols, greens such as Romaine lettuce, spinach, and chard.
Effect: Increases Vata, reduces Pitta, reduces Kapha. Most bitter foods are stimulants and promote digestion and cleanse the blood.

AYURVEDIC EATING FOR YOUR METABOLIC TYPE

VATA

Vata people should aim to stick to salty, sour and sweet tasting foods, and oily foods to maintain balance. They should also attempt to eat at regular intervals.

Vegetables

Sweet potatoes, cooked tomatoes, onion, okra, cooked spinach, pumpkin, green beans, courgettes, artichokes, asparagus, cucumbers, leeks, carrots, garlic, black olives, cooked peas, radishes, green chillies, beets, watercress.

Grains and seeds

Rice, sesame seeds, sunflower seeds, wheat, pumpkin seeds, cooked oats, quinoa.

Fruit

Generally, most sweet fruits: melons, mangoes, apples, papaya, bananas, avocado, grapes, apricots, dates, fresh figs, lemons, limes, oranges, strawberries, berries, pineapple.

Meat and fish

Chicken, duck, beef, turkey, shellfish in moderation. *Vatas* benefit particularly from eating plenty of meat and fish.

Beans and pulses

Red lentils, mung beans, mung daal, urad daal.

Dairy produce

Cows' and goats' milk, cheese and cottage cheese, eggs, ghee, yoghurt. All dairy is good for *Vatas* in moderate quantities.

Herbs and spices

Fresh ginger, mint, paprika, nutmeg, peppermint, thyme, turmeric, dill, fennel, cloves, coriander, cardamom, black mustard, basil, cumin, oregano, vanilla and parsley.

Others

Cashews, brazil nuts, pine nuts, pecans, walnuts, pistachios, almonds, coconut, sesame oil, spicy tea, warm drinks, fresh fruit and vegetable juices, herbal teas: camomile, fennel, fenugreek, elderflower, fresh ginger, lemon grass, juniper berry, licorice.

KAPHA

Kapha types respond best to warming foods, and so should aim to eat cooked meals rather than cold and raw foods.

Vegetables

Cabbage, Brussels sprouts, carrots, cauliflower, cooked peas, peppers, swede, watercress, turnips, sweetcorn, mushrooms, green beans, okra, black olives, cooked onions, parsnip, garlic, cucumber, leeks, sweet potatoes, pumpkin.

Grains and seeds

Pumpkin and sunflower seeds (toasted), polenta, popcorn, oatbran, couscous, buckwheat, corn, barley, rye.

Fruit

Generally, most astringent fruits; cranberries, peaches, raisins, cherries, pears, pomegranates, prunes, apples.

Meat and fish
Freshwater fish, turkey, venison, eggs, shrimps, rabbit, chicken.

Beans and pulses
Black eyed beans, chick peas, brown and red lentils, mung beans, mung daal, soy beans, tempeh, tofu, white beans, black beans.

Dairy produce
Low fat cows' milk or soya milk.

Herbs and spices
Ginger, garlic, mustard, onions, parsley, any hot spices, chilli pepper, black pepper, coriander, horseradish.

Others
Mustard/safflower/sunflower oils, mango juice, carrot juice, any vegetable juice, grape juice, cranberry juice, spicy teas, herbal teas: cinnamon, clove, dandelion, chamomile, blackberry, alfalfa, catnip.

PITTA
Pitta type people should avoid all spicy, fried, hot and sour foods since these will aggravate the dosha. This body type is hot, so you should eat cooling, refreshing foods, especially in the summer – raw rather than cooked foods and vegetarian for preference.

Vegetables
Peas, potatoes, onions, mushrooms, green peppers, cauliflower, Brussels sprouts, asparagus, artichokes, broccoli, squash, cabbage, carrots, cucumbers, courgettes, fennel, celery, green beans, leeks, lettuce, spinach, black olives, leafy greens.

Grains and seeds
Basmati rice, flax seeds, barley, rice cakes, sunflower seeds, white rice, wheat.

Fruit
Generally, most sweet fruits: pineapple, ripe mangoes, plums and apricots, berries and cherries, pomegranate, pears, grapes, melons, dates, figs; apples, avocado.

Meat and fish
Freshwater fish, rabbit, turkey, chicken.

Beans and pulses
Chickpeas, kidney beans, lentils, lima beans, mung beans, mung daal, soya beans, tofu, white beans, black beans.

Dairy produce
Yoghurt, ghee, goats' milk, unsalted butter, cottage cheese, soft cheeses, cows' milk.

Herbs and spices
Fresh ginger, cinnamon, basil, fennel, mint, cumin, dill, aloe vera, coriander.

Others
Almonds, coconuts, most fresh fruit juices, herbal teas: dandelion, camomile, chicory, alfalfa, catnip, elderflower, jasmine, fennel, fresh ginger, blackberry.

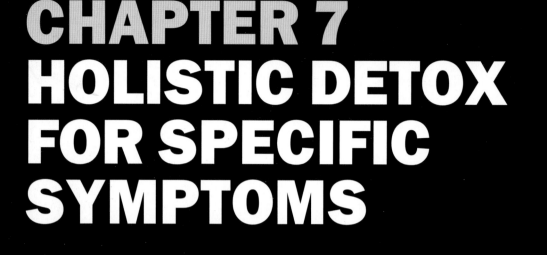

CHAPTER 7
HOLISTIC DETOX FOR SPECIFIC SYMPTOMS

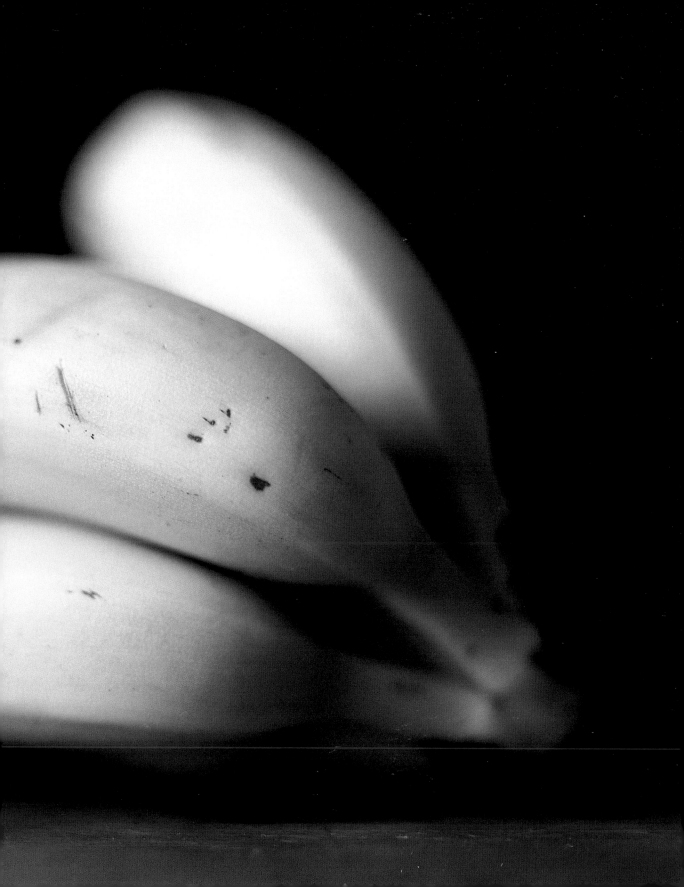

EVERYTHING WE EAT AFFECTS OUR PHYSICAL, MENTAL AND EMOTIONAL HEALTH. THIS CHAPTER SHOWS YOU HOW, BY BUILDING ON WHAT YOU HAVE LEARNED USING THE SELF-DIAGNOSIS TOOLS IN THE PREVIOUS CHAPTER AND ADAPTING THE MAINTENANCE PROGRAMME, YOU CAN REDUCE YOUR DEPENDENCE ON PRESCRIPTION MEDICATION AND ERADICATE YOUR HEADACHES, CONSTIPATION, BLOATING AND MOOD SWINGS – TO NAME BUT A HANDFUL OF COMMON SYMPTOMS. I AM NOT TALKING ABOUT ALL MEDICATION OF COURSE. THOSE SUFFERING SERIOUS CONDITIONS HAVE, I AM AFRAID, TO CONTINUE WITH THEIR PRESCRIPTION DRUGS. BUT I STRONGLY ADVISE THAT THOSE OF YOU ON CHOLESTEROL MEDICATION, THYROID-GLAND PRESCRIPTION DRUGS, BLOOD- PRESSURE PILLS AND HRT, SHOULD CONSULT YOUR PHYSICIAN BEFORE STARTING THE DETOX PROGRAMME AND VISIT AGAIN AT THE END OF THE 21-DAY PERIOD TO SEE HOW YOUR PRESCRIPTION PROFILE HAS CHANGED. HOPEFULLY, ANY AILMENT WILL HAVE BECOME LESS OF AN ISSUE.

JOINT ACHES AND PAINS

If you suffer from muscle tension – your legs often tight and tired, shoulders stiff and back a bit achy – then you are one of the many people who suffer from musculoskeletal fibro-myalgia, a medical term for pain within the muscle. Reports estimate that 80 per cent of the population will suffer from lower-back pain at some point in their lives, and the other 20 per cent will suffer from neck pain, so you are almost bound to suffer a musculoskeletal ache at some point! Why? We are all becoming more sedentary; working longer hours; experiencing heightened mental anxieties; driving everywhere and taking little or no exercise and having a poor diet – a great recipe for muscle tension and stiffness.

You probably don't always register how miserable your muscles are. Sometimes, the clue only comes when having a neck or shoulder massage feels so painful and sensitive that you suddenly realise how tight and knotted your muscles have become. The body is able to desensitise itself and can block the messages that the shoulders are trying to send to the brain. That is why it is imperative to address muscular skeletal aches and pains whenever you notice them so they don't cause bigger problems later.

Extending the muscular tissues, by taking more exercise and stretching regularly, will improve blood flow and loosen those stiff areas. You will probably be well aware of the detoxing benefits of stretching during exercise and going to a steam room or sauna where the heat encourages the muscles to relax and the blood to flow better (followed, of course, by drinking plenty of water).

Adopting a more alkaline diet neutralises the build up of lactic acids within the muscles, while releasing the tightness in your muscles frees the bottlenecking of all the toxins that have become entrapped and embedded in your tissues, thus allowing those toxins to be released and flushed out of your system.

These are only small changes but, if you take the time to incorporate them into your life, you will be helping to prevent the onset of chronic illnesses.

BLOATING

Bloating is an enlargement or distension of the stomach. It's not necessarily the fat that's contained in the stomach itself, but more probably a swelling of the abdomen that's mainly caused by eating a lot of gassy foods. It can also be a result of increased water within the digestive system. People who suffer from bloating usually also complain of passing a lot of wind, being quite flatulent and burping a lot.

If you are prone to bloating, you should obviously avoid gas-forming foods such as raw vegetables and salads, and beans such as chickpeas, baked beans, kidney beans, and fizzy drinks. Try and stick to steamed green vegetables and stir-fries, where possible, instead of salads. Over a period of time, as the bloating subsides, you can gradually reintroduce them back into your system, taking care to make them an occasional treat rather than an everyday staple. Sugary foods can also be gas forming because they ferment with your gut bacteria and any candida you may have. The resulting gas can lead to bloating plus uncomfortable wind and flatulence.

HEADACHES

As we all know there are a variety of different types of headaches. You may get one because you are not controlling blood sugar levels or because you've been staring at your computer screen all day (probably an 'eye-strain' headache). The clue to their type usually lies in where they occur (for example, on one side of the head or above the eye(s) or on both sides of the head) and at what frequency. It is vitally important that you consult your GP if you suffer from recurrent headaches and are not sure what is causing them. It is essential to understand their cause rather than masking the symptoms by taking painkillers. You may be anaesthetising the painful effects of a more serious condition.

If, however, you suffer from the occasional mild headache or even from migraine, there are lots of things you can try to alleviate the pain. If your headaches occur when you feel hungry or have missed a meal, it could be that you have a low sugar tolerance. Some of my patients find that, if they haven't eaten enough or they've gone for a long time without eating, they will get a low-blood-sugar headache.

Many headaches are due to dehydration. This will be worsened by working in an air-conditioned environment. Check that you are drinking your couple of litres of water a day as an alternative to grabbing the aspirin or the ibuprofen.

If you get headaches that affect your vision, they are more likely to be migraines. Make sure that your glasses are the right prescription, or have an eye test. There are umpteen remedies out there for migraines, but check, first, whether yours might be food related. You may have an allergy to chocolate, or coffee, or to acid-forming foods. Consult the Alkaline and Acid Foods list in Chapter 3 and avoid the acid-forming nasties as much as possible.

WEIGHT PROBLEMS

Checking with the Body Mass Index chart will have left you much clearer about the ideal weight for your body type and height, and whether you are (or have been) overweight. The Holistic Detox isn't focussed purely on losing weight, but it is certainly true that one by-product of the Programme is weight loss. Far better, however, to focus on improved energy levels, better skin complexion, less bloating etc. Everyone knows that diets geared to losing weight do not work. The reason my Holistic Detox Programme does work is because its focus is on improving our health and environment. Changing certain elements of your dietary habits, and reducing the effects of chemicals, preservatives and refined foods in your diet, will have dramatic results.

As your body detoxes, you are automatically going to start shedding weight. If you want to lose more, you should aim to prolong the Detox Programme to four or six weeks for maximum benefit. Then you can move on to a six-week maintenance period. See how you feel. Monitor your progress and don't forget that, if you begin to suffer any unpleasant side effects, stop immediately and seek advice from your GP.

JULIETTE'S STORY

I had been feeling below par for quite a while. A few years ago, I had bronchitis, which ran into bronchial pneumonia; and then, last year, I contracted bronchitis again and just couldn't shake it off. It wasn't that I still felt ill as such – I just didn't feel well. Something wasn't quite right.

Twenty years ago, I had a hysterectomy and that led me to put on three stone in weight. It was obviously a substantial amount and I think it's fair to say that turned me into a different person. For years, I'd been trying different diets and going to Weight Watchers. It was always the same. I would shift a stone, put it back on again, then go back through the whole routine, and so on – but I never managed to get back to the weight I had been before I had the operation.

Before I went to see Joshi, I was taking thyroxin for an under-active thyroid. I had recently been on HRT and was self-administering vitamin pills in a bid to increase my energy levels. I did go to the gym to try and keep fit but my knee kept hurting, which hampered me a bit. Basically, I just wasn't firing on all cylinders.

Then, last April, I read an article about Joshi and decided to go and see him. He was like a breath of fresh air. He didn't tell me I was fat or make me feel depressed. He just took my pulse, checked my tongue and spent a long time talking to me. He produced a diet for me to follow and I began it that same evening.

The next day, I felt quite grotty and the day after that I got a terrible migraine. I called him and said that I didn't feel very well. He told me that my reaction was normal and that, in fact, it meant that I was getting better because the toxins were at last being released and were entering my bloodstream. It was true. Within a few days I felt fantastic.

I only lost one pound the first week, then three pounds in the second week and two pounds in the third week. But the extraordinary thing was that I didn't even feel like I was trying to lose the weight. I honestly didn't notice. Within four weeks I'd lost 10 lbs. I carried on for three months and lost 22lbs. I'm not consciously on a diet any more, but I've changed the way I eat and am confident that I will lose more weight just because I do things differently now.

I never found the diet a problem, not even in the first few weeks. It's easy once you get going. At first I was worried that I would miss caffeine –I do like my Starbuck café lattes – and I love shellfish! In fact, I haven't missed either of those things. I did wonder, the other day, what it would be like to have some lobster but, to be honest, I'm not even sure if I'd like it any more. Strangely, the only thing I really miss is balsamic vinegar.

The programme has helped to get my blood pressure back to normal (it had been very low before) and I've been able to stop taking my thyroxin tablets. I had stopped taking HRT, just before I went to see Joshi, because I had read that it is bad for you, but I was very worried about how I would cope. In fact, I haven't missed it all.

Because Joshi had removed all citrus fruits from my diet, my knee stopped hurting and I was able to go back to the gym. I've gone down a dress size and a half and everyone keeps telling me how amazing I look.

I feel better than I have in years. It's not just about weight but about my whole sense of wellbeing.

MRS JULIETTE FARQHAR, 55, RUNS HER OWN PR AGENCY – 'JULIETTE HELLMAN'. SHE LIVES IN LONDON WITH HER TWO CHILDREN.

SKIN CONDITIONS

If you are prone to eczema, psoriasis, spots or acne, or find that you are, pre-menopause, growing excess facial hair, it could be that your problems are nutrition-related. Acne in mature women can be the result of a hormonal imbalance due to cysts on their ovaries (which has nutritional implications). A sallow skin could be the result of an iron deficiency and liver congestion. Look at the colour of your skin and eyes. If you have a yellowish complexion, it may that you are a little jaundiced in which case your liver could be diseased. If you feel even slightly alarmed, consult your GP.

Skin conditions such as psoriasis, dermatitis and eczema are often aggravated by stress and the advice on meditation and yoga in Chapter 8 is particularly useful for people suffering from skin problems since it promotes relaxation. But how many people realise that their skin can also become inflamed through eating too much sugar, wine, or acidic foods? One of the main homeopathic cures given to these sufferers is sulphur. Sulphur is contained in dark green vegetables (such as kale, spinach, broccoli, cabbage, and greens) and these help the liver purify the blood. As it purifies, it rids the body of toxins and acidities and that, in turn, improves the skin's elasticity and complexion. In this way, the condition that produces these skin problems is eliminated. Don't rely on trying to improve your complexion through using expensive face creams and skin preparations. Often, having an internal spring clean can have a dramatic effect on your skin complexion, colour, tone, feel and elasticity – you really are what you eat.

If you are prone to spots, flaky skin, blotchiness, irritations and eruptions, you need to avoid sugars, particularly refined sugars and acidic foods and fruits such as oranges and grapefruit. Steer clear of alcohol too, especially wine, beer and champagne. Fizzy drinks will also increase acidity and make sensitive skins itch.

Many eczema sufferers find that, every time they have cakes, biscuits or chocolate, their skin becomes redder, itchier and more inflamed. Understand that a lot of allergic dermatitis can be a result of the body's inability to cope with chemicals.

Beware of medicated skin preparations. A lot of people experience unpleasant reactions so check the label or ask a pharmacist to decipher it for you. Other creams, liquids and lotions can irritate skin, such as cleansing agents, hair mousses, gels, dyes, perfumes and shampoos. They are full of toxins that your liver is too overworked to process, and so their poisons end up in your bloodstream.

Rather than force your poor body to deal with the allergic and toxic response that resulted in a skin condition – look after your liver! In place of that mid-morning chocolate bar, have some organic carrot sticks. Try to avoid the refined 'killer' sugars and stick to rice syrup, molasses and honey. See if you still get the same reaction. Try alternatives one at a time: for example, first try the honey, then the maple syrup and then rice syrup. All of these are good natural products.

As an alternative to dairy produce, which can also produce dermatitis or eczema, try soya milk. Avoid goats' and sheep's milk as they can have the same effects as cows' milk. Feta cheese, ricotta and even, to an extent, buffalo mozzarella should also be avoided. As an alternative to potatoes and tomatoes, stick to green vegetables, either steaming them, or stir-frying. Think about having more fresh salads, too, adding kidney beans, pulses and lentils. Vary your salads so you don't get bored with them.

TIREDNESS AND LETHARGY

Tiredness, lethargy or fatigue can be described as an inability to perform all the required physical and mental demands we put on ourselves (within reason). Remember, rest is vital for optimum health. Listen to your body, rest when you need to, even if it means occasionally curtailing your social life.

If you feel that you're struggling with everyday activities – for instance, if you frequently wake up in the morning feeling sluggish and are then unable to concentrate on the challenges that are thrown at you – I would say that you are suffering from significant tiredness.

We are usually aware, when we're tired, of why we are tired and the kind of tiredness we are experiencing. We know when we are healthily or physically tired, as when after a nice long walk, a couple of hours of tennis, or a day's retail therapy. However, if this weariness is as a result of sleep deprivation or mental stress – or even after eating certain foods – then we know we are experiencing an unhealthy feeling of lethargy and irritability.

If you are prone to 'unhealthy' lethargy, make sure that you are drinking adequate levels of water to keep your blood pressure up. Avoid the yo-yo effects of eating refined sugars that destabilise your blood-sugar levels, and eliminate dairy foods because they can encourage the body to produce high levels of tryptophan, a hormone that can induce lethargy. These foods also require a lot of energy to digest, as does red meat.

Really try to reduce your stress levels as much as possible and find other ways of dealing with your pent up feelings than drinking alcohol or smoking, perhaps through exercise, yoga, meditation or taking up an all-consuming interest such as painting or music. Although it may seem counterintuitive, increasing physical exercise – using a treadmill or taking a bike ride or a swim – may well boost your energy levels because exercise increases your metabolic rate. It encourages your body to produce endorphins – natural hormones that make you feel good and more energised.

To boost your energy levels, you need to avoid energy-sapping foods such as bread, biscuits, dairy produce, cakes, chocolate and alcohol, which are all going to make you more tired. Drinking large amounts of alcohol is particularly tiring because its initial effect on the body – as a stimulant hitting the central nervous system with a sudden injection of sugar – wears off. Indeed, as the body starts metabolising the alcohol, you will probably start to feel tired and dehydrated because, as you eliminate the liquid from your body, you also eliminate many essential minerals and salts. When feeling hung-over the next day, therefore, as well as drinking lots of water, you would do well to eat a banana, which, being full of potassium and magnesium, can replace some of the minerals you have expelled. Your body will respond very quickly, after the minerals have been replaced, and those morning-after symptoms will soon be gone.

Banish your tiredness with energy-giving foods – raw vegetables, raw juices, plenty of water, bananas, fresh chicken, fish, nuts, pulses, grains and freshly prepared foods. They are full of vitality and allow your body to absorb their ample nutrients without taxing your digestive system. They will, therefore, reach your essential organs more quickly.

CONSTIPATION

People are more constipated than they realise. I've always been fascinated with the fact that people think that having one bowel movement a day, or even every other day, is normal when they're eating three or four meals a day. First we have breakfast; then at around eleven we have a mid-morning snack; a few hours later we have lunch; at about four we have some tea and biscuits and then we have supper. We will probably have a pee several times during the day, but only go to the loo properly the following morning, and just the once. We may have taken, perhaps, three or four – or sometimes five – meals and snacks throughout the day. This means that the food and resulting waste matter and toxins are putrefying within our digestive system, giving us bloating, flatulence and wind, and making us feel heavy, sluggish and lethargic – and we are surprised!

The trouble is that constipation allows the excess waste to remain within our body for a long period of time. It has to be dealt with and we have to encourage the elimination processes within the body to work at an adequate level so that we are going to the loo three or four times a day. In this way, as we are taking in food, we are digesting it, processing it and eliminating the waste as efficiently as possible.

One of the aims of the Holistic Detox Programme is to allow your body to maintain normal gut mobility. To achieve this, you have to avoid constipation. This means avoiding glutinous foods that, literally, glue themselves to the wall of your gut. One effective way is to reduce dairy produce and red meat as these can be difficult to digest. Additionally, you should eat more fibrous foods, more gluten-free cereals, green vegetables and salads, and drink plenty of water to keep your food hydrated so that it doesn't become dry and stick to the gut wall.

If you're a persistent constipation sufferer, you should incorporate into the 21-Day Detox Programme a gentle laxative such as senna.

INDIGESTION

Indigestion, as the name suggests, is the body's inability to digest food and process the nutrients, fats, acids and other constituent elements. You know you're suffering from indigestion when you get heartburn. Heartburn is that feeling, after you've eaten something, of discomfort around the upper part of the digestive system where the stomach is, just under the ribcage. It may be that food is perhaps stuck here. There's that feeling of being much more full than normal and, when you lie down, a burning sensation (see below under Heartburn). It can also occur lower down in your digestive system, for which there can be several causes. It could be the inability of your body to digest the food that you've have eaten, which happens quite often with meat which is rich in protein and takes the body a long time to break down. Similar problems arise with dairy produce and with alcohol and fruit. It can also be caused by increased acidity within the gut, eating food too quickly and overloading the system, producing too much gas, or because of a block within the digestive tract from dry foods or, perhaps, even a spasm within your digestive musculature.

Recognise the foods that give you indigestion and the frequency of the attacks. They may take the form of heartburn or of a pain in the stomach that occurs before eating, or after eating or at different times of the day. If it happens often and does not respond to changing your diet, I would urge you to consult your physician rather than masking the symptoms with antacid.

HEARTBURN

Heartburn is often experienced after eating foods that produce too much acid within the stomach. When food is swallowed and taken into the stomach, there is a little valve that shuts and closes allowing the food to be digested within the stomach itself. Sometimes the acids which are produced in the stomach to digest protein can irritate this valve and allow it to open slightly. The result is a slight reflux of acid that enters the oesophagus (the food pipe) and causes discomfort. This condition is known as a hiatus hernia.

Heartburn patients are recommended to avoid a lot of sugary and dairy foods. Spicy and fried foods can also produce heartburn, as can beer, fermented foods, and, of course, red meat and sugar. So, eliminating these foods as much as possible will reduce the symptoms of heartburn and lead to a less painful digestive experience.

Recurrent heartburn can be the result of taking too many painkillers, so recognise the effects of these and consult your physician accordingly. He/she may recommend that you take an antacid that will reduce the amount of acid produced within your stomach. But the top priority is to avoid the acid-forming foods in the first place.

INSOMNIA

Insomnia is failure to get a good night's sleep – either because you experience interrupted sleep throughout the night, or because you can't get to sleep. This condition may be caused by stress or anxiety which leads to remaining alert at night.

Somebody who isn't getting enough sleep (ideally between seven and eight hours a night), or has difficulty getting to sleep (and thus trouble waking up in the morning) may be considered an insomniac. The ideal night's rest is when you fall asleep quite quickly and wake up in the morning feeling refreshed, invigorated and rested. If you are not one of these people, then perhaps you're an insomniac.

Certain foods can exacerbate insomnia, including dairy produce. Eating very late at night is also a no-no as the still-undigested food in your stomach can make you feel heavy, bloated and full – which encourages insomnia. Although people regard alcohol as a relaxant, it can disrupt sleep patterns and affect our central nervous system therefore encouraging insomnia. Stimulants such as alcohol, caffeine, coffee or tea, if drunk after about 6pm, can over-stimulate the body at a time when it should be winding down.

If you suffer from sleep problems, do some exercises that will use up all that mental and physical energy stored in your body. Try some yoga to stretch and loosen up your muscles and relax your body, or some gentle breathing and meditation exercises to relax your mind. Reading a few pages of a book (providing it is not a murder mystery!) can also help you drift off. If you are worried about a big day ahead, then write your concerns on a piece of paper and leave it on the bedside table, rather than taking your worries to bed.

Certain herbal, caffeine-free teas, such as camomile, are an ideal bedtime tonic for an insomniac as they help the body relax. If you have difficulty relaxing for long periods of time, then take a herbal supplement, such as valerian or rhodiola, which will help your body establish normal sleep patterns.

MOOD SWINGS

Mood swings can be regarded as a change in our psychological attitude to certain situations. For example, you may find that all of a sudden, and for no reason, you suddenly feel agitated, anxious or irritable. If your blood sugar levels drop suddenly, this biochemical change within your body may leave you feeling irritable. Normally, the quick-fix solution would be to grab a chocolate bar in order to feel calmer again.

These mood swings need to be recognised and addressed. We have to realise that, if they are the result of some sort of imbalance – low blood-sugar levels, drinking too much coffee – we can sort these out ourselves. What we put in our bodies can alter our psychological make up.

If you are prone to mood swings and changes in your personality as a result of certain foods or drinks, recognise this – and lay off them. Substitute sugar-free muesli bars, raw vegetables, freshly filtered water and ripe bananas for the alcohol, sugar, cake, biscuits and chocolate.

Alcohol in particular is often misused as a prop to deal with mood swings, but people who drink alcohol on a daily basis are often prone to chronic depression. One of the reasons for this is that alcohol depletes the liver of B vitamins which are necessary to maintain good neural and mental health. So avoid those bars after work where you might drink so much wine or beer that you become too tired to have an evening meal. Instead, encourage social interaction with your friends at a favourite restaurant where you can sit down with some grilled chicken or steamed fish, fresh vegetables and a vodka with cranberry juice. You can still have a good night out, but without the toxic side effects of a night's bingeing which will, inevitably, affect your mood in a negative way.

Many women, around the time of their menstrual period, find that they get very weepy and emotional. They don't feel in control, they may be forgetful, drop things and behave clumsily. These symptoms of teariness or irritation can be very frustrating and all too often see people reaching for a quick fix. It is far more constructive, though, to rely on healthy snacks and herbal teas than chocolate or cakes.

Drinking too much coffee can trigger a mood swing provoked by the caffeine – and you may not even be aware of the cause if you drink a lot. And don't forget that many foods that are processed and packaged and available on our supermarket shelves will be poison to mood-swing sufferers if they contain a lot of additives and preservatives. Begin to monitor your mood swings, which may also be having quite a profound effect on those around you. Recognise the symptoms and ask those close to you for feedback about when and how you get irritable, boisterous or even aggressive. Then, you need to relate your mood swings to your diet and recognise that you may have to cut down your alcohol intake, your addiction to sugar, or a dependency on caffeine.

If you recognise that you suffer from extreme mood swings, and they are having a debilitating affect on your life, you should consult your physician. His/her advice, combined with your effort in cutting out aggravating foods, will help re-establish equilibrium and harmony in your life.

CHAPTER 8
USING COMPLEMENTARY THERAPIES

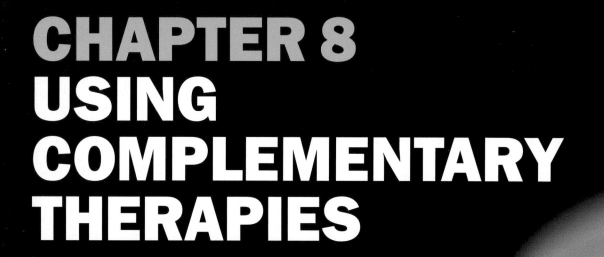

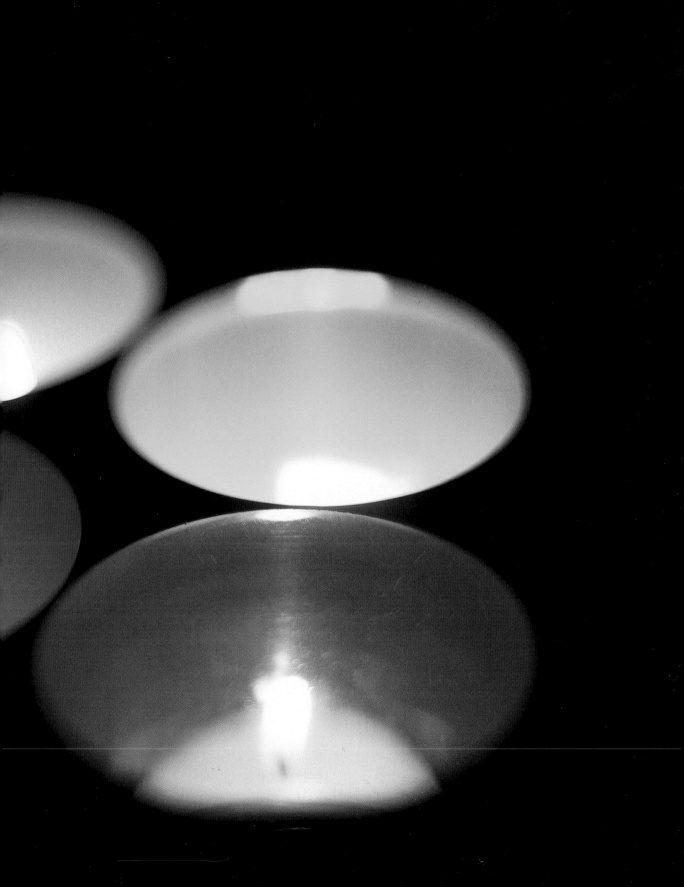

THOSE OF YOU WHO NEED A LITTLE EXTRA HELP GETTING YOUR BODY TO RESPOND TO THE HOLISTIC DETOX MORE EFFICIENTLY OR QUICKLY MAY LIKE TO CONSIDER SOME OF THE FOLLOWING TRIED AND TESTED THERAPIES AND EXERCISES. I PRESCRIBE MANY OF THESE TO MY PATIENTS WHO MANIFEST SUCH CONDITIONS AS DIGESTION PROBLEMS, ALLERGIES, STRESS AILMENTS OR MUSCULAR DISCOMFORT. YOU CAN FIND A LIST OF EXPERIENCED PRACTITIONERS AND WEBSITES IN THE DIRECTORY ON PAGE 188 BUT IF YOU CANNOT FIND ONE NEAR YOU, ASK YOUR GP. MANY NHS SURGERIES NOW HAVE ALTERNATIVE PRACTITIONERS BASED WITH THEM. IF NOT, HE OR SHE MAY SURPRISE YOU AND RECOMMEND ONE!

ACUPUNCTURE

Acupuncture is an ancient Chinese technique in which hair-thin needles are inserted into specific points on the body to prevent or treat disease.

According to traditional Eastern philosophy, our health and wellbeing entirely depends on the body's energy flow – or qi (pronounced chi).

Qi is the vital life force that moves, protects, transforms and warms everything in our body. It travels via 14 primary pathways or meridians and is also made of two equal and opposite qualities – yin and yang. When yin and yang are in harmony, qi flows freely within these channels and a person is well. If they become unbalanced the meridians can become blocked, resulting in ill health. The flow of qi can be disturbed by a number of factors including anxiety, stress, poor nutrition, infections, even the weather.

To strengthen the flow of qi or remove blockages in the meridians, an acupuncturist inserts a number of tiny, sterile needles just under the skin at certain specific points. Otherwise known as acupoints, there are four to five hundred of them along the energy pathways and each one is associated with specific areas of the body.

For instance, if you are suffering from nausea, needles might be inserted into points on your wrist while a vision problem might be treated with needles in the foot. There are as many as two hundred of these points in the outer ear alone and they all relate to a different area of our anatomy such as the knees, hips, liver and heart. Acting a little like a switchboard to the brain, each acupoint, when treated, triggers electrical impulses via the brain to the corresponding point in the body.

The aim is to stimulate the body's own healing response and help restore its natural balance.

As is typical of Chinese remedies, acupuncture takes a holistic approach and practitioners will address the matter of spiritual and emotional equilibrium, as much as the physical, in their treatments and diagnoses.

Many people are frightened by acupuncture because they are worried about the needles but they are not at all like the household ones we are familiar with. They are very flexible and almost thread-like (only about three times the thickness of a human hair). And while they can feel uncomfortable at times, they are designed to enter the skin with little resistance and rarely hurt. Most people usually describe a tingling feeling or, at the very most, a slight ache.

Anything from one to 15 needles are used. They are inserted to a depth of 13 – 25 mm depending on the location of the acupoint and are left in for anything from a few seconds to 40 minutes depending on the treatment.

Acupuncture can be used during the Holistic Detox to stimulate certain meridians or energy channels to improve the function of the organ they correspond to. It is almost like turning up or turning down the dimmer switch to your lights – you can stimulate or calm down the area of dysfunction, for example your liver, and thus encourage balance and a more harmonious and healthy body. I quite often use ear acupuncture to control cravings and to help regulate blood sugar levels. I place small ear needles on specific points, which helps to suppress the patient's cravings for chocolate, for example, or alcohol. It is also very effective in helping people to stop smoking.

ALLERGY ELIMINATION

An allergy arises when the immune system develops a hypersensitive reaction to a food or substance. Eliminating an allergy first requires diagnosing which food or group of foods the patient may be allergic to. At the first consultation the therapist will take details and find out to which foods the patient believes he reacts negatively, what those reactions are and how long he has experienced them. The major foods and food groups to which people find they are allergic are those containing gluten, dairy and wheat, which is why I recommend avoiding these completely on the 21-Day Detox and introducing them gradually and carefully in the maintenance phase of the Holistic Detox. Simply following my plan may be enough to eliminate allergies that arise from a sluggish digestive system but others can be more intransigent and require specific treatment.

The most common reactions a patient manifests after eating foods to which he is allergic include skin irritations, sinusitis, congestion and headaches. The most serious reaction is Anaphylactic shock, when the patient's body goes into spasm or his throat swells so he cannot breathe, which can be life-threatening and requires hospital treatment. This can happen if the person has a peanut allergy or as a result of a bee or wasp sting.

The aim of an allergy therapist is to identify the culprit food group or groups and clear the body of the reaction. After the allergy has been detected and treated the patient must avoid that food for 24 hours. Some stubborn allergies may take several treatments before they are eliminated. In my view, the most effective allergy eliminators use the Nambudripad allergy elimination technique known as NAET, which involves first testing the patient for allergies to the major food groups using kinesiology (a muscle testing technique to detect functional imbalances in the body) and then a treatment on the back based on Chinese acupressure (acupuncture without needles that relies on touch). The idea of this treatment is to open up the patient's energy channels while he is holding a phial of the elements he is allergic to. The treatment is gentle, painless and non-invasive and extremely effective in that it can permanently eliminate allergies.

Major food allergens

Egg group – which includes chicken, feathers, tetracycline in antibiotics found in chicken.

Calcium – milk, cheese, uncooked dark leaf vegetables, sardines, salmon, sunflower seeds.

Vitamin C – fruit, vegetables, dry fruit, soft drinks, milk, artificial sweeteners.

Vitamin B-Complex – whole grain products including wheat, bread, flour.

Sugar – all processed foods, chocolate and candy, fruit.

Iron mix – apricots, dates, bananas, broccoli, lentils, egg yolk, liver, red meat, spinach and chocolate.

Vitamin A – fish, shellfish, fruits and vegetables.

Mineral mix – mineral water, root vegetables such as onions, potatoes, carrots, turnips and metallic objects such as taps and cooking equipment.

Salt mix and chlorides – kelp, celery, seafood, lettuce, all processed foods, dried and cured meats, ham, bacon and kidneys.

Food intolerance

Intolerance arises in similar ways to allergies and is treated using the principles of elimination and gradual and moderate reintroduction. A typical example of food intolerance is to have a migraine reaction when you drink orange juice, but not every time. For example, I am unable to drink orange juice in this country but in India I am fine. This is because the juice there is purely organic, produced using only natural fertilisers and no pesticides; I obviously have an intolerance to the pesticide present in orange juice sold in this country rather than an allergy to oranges.

People develop food intolerances mainly through exposure to unnatural chemicals, colourants and additives. But the body can also develop an intolerance to certain foods due to it becoming over-sensitised. For example, years ago I used to eat pistachio nuts by the kilo. On one particularly holiday I would sit with my father on the beach every evening and work my way through a two kilo bag of pistachios. Several months later I had a few pistachios again and suddenly developed a terrible rash on my back and face. I had over-sensitised my body to the nuts by 'overdosing' on them over a period of time, so for a long time afterwards even when I ate just a few, the condition became inflamed and the body shouted stop. Elimination and careful reintroduction has been effective in eliminating this intolerance.

BEVERLEY'S STORY

Since seeing the effects of Joshi's Holistic Detox, my husband now tells his friends, 'Don't get a mistress, get a Joshi wife'. There I was, mother of three, approaching 49 and suffering grumbling stomach pains, bloated, lethargic and unable to lose weight. My GP had given me tablets that had the terrible side effects of giving me panic attacks and shortness of breath. I had given up smoking over 20 a day and put on a stone. I was also suffering hot flushes, night sweats and mood swings.

My GP put me on HRT but I still had no energy. Then I read about Dr Joshi's Holistic Detox and thought I would make the effort and go to London to see him. Forty-eight hours after going on his diet, I was feeling better. I was 11 stone 8lb when I first went to see him and am now 10 stone 1lb.

As well as following the Programme, I had some colonic irrigation – I was a bit nervous about that – but it was fantastic. I realised that dairy products are like a poison to me and that yeast is no good either, yet my doctor had prescribed yeast to ease my leg cramps. Joshi got me off that and also threw away my HRT. He made me feel like I was 30 again. No more hot sweats, flushes or cramps, and the best thing of all was that he cured my cellulite! I am back to wearing mini skirts and everyone is saying how fantastic I look – including my husband.

Now, I don't take any supplements but just stick to his Detox as much as I can. No red meat, yeast or dairy products. My bottom and legs are not quite like Claudia Schiffer's, but they are not bad – and so much better than before. My skin is smoother and my weight is stable. I have no upset stomach, more energy and am sleeping better – and all because I have got rid of the poisons in my system.

BEVERLEY YOUNG 49, MOTHER OF THREE FROM LEIGHTON BUZZARD.

ENDOMOLOGY

Endomology is a non surgical cosmetic procedure which helps to reduce cellulite and fat through an intensive massage performed by a machine. The machine comprises a system of rollers which when operated by an experienced therapist can help to shift fat in stubborn areas and improve lymphatic draining through a suction device thus helping to remove toxins from the body. This treatment is an excellent complement to the Holistic Detox as it works on stimulating the fat layers just beneath the skin encouraging them to break down and drain the fluid out of the body. Women typically have four fat layers compared to men who only have three, which is why they tend to have more of it and find it hard to shift. The fatty area women find the most stubborn is the subcutaneous fat layer, a mere six millimetres deep and just below the surface of the skin. Endomology softens and loosens this fatty area which is typically very prone to cellulite and stimulates circulation by flushing toxins from the body and thereby improving blood supply. Recommended treatment is 35–40 minutes twice a week for five weeks.

There is no registered body or association for endomologists. This treatment is not yet widely available so ask your local homeopath or GP for advice.

HYPNOTHERAPY

Hypnotherapy is a non-invasive alternative treatment for people who want to generate change in their lives but need some help and mental support. It could be that we feel stuck because we can't let go of a relationship from which we need to release ourselves or that we are comfort eating because we have never properly grieved for a family member or friend who has died. We may not know the reason for a lot of the bad habits we want to be rid of. The hypnotherapist is there to cleanse the recesses of our mind by ridding it of the stored toxic debris that is poisoning our chances of happiness. Hypnotherapy is particularly complementary to the Holistic Detox if you are struggling with giving up particular foodstuffs such as chocolate, for example. It helps us achieve what we desire through reinforcing and bolstering us by tapping into our subconscious, a huge reservoir of power through which we can be motivated to make radical changes.

We all get bogged down with emotional stuff now and again and in just the same way that we need to cleanse our bodies, we need to detox our emotional system and banish the debris from our head in order to recover a sense of reality that is balanced rather than distorted. A hypnotherapist helps achieve this firstly by talking to the patient to discover what he wants to achieve and why, and then relaxing him in order to tap into the unconscious part of the mind. Harnessing the power of suggestion by using simple language and positive focus, the therapist helps to initiate the change their patient wants to make so that it becomes as automatic as brushing their teeth.

The results can be dramatic – it is possible to cure patients of their desire to smoke in one session – but other problems may take longer to address. A serious commitment to change is always crucial.

MASSAGE AND REFLEXOLOGY

Massage is an excellent way of stimulating the blood to flow around the body. The various massage techniques are designed to disperse any build up of deoxygenated blood or lactic acid toxins in the muscles which may be causing pain and stress. A bundle of knots which we recognise as pain and tension, and commonly gather in the back, neck and shoulders can be untangled with deep massage so that fresh oxygenated blood can pass through and nourish the muscle enabling it to work properly. Massage can be particularly useful for people on the Holistic Detox as some people experience muscle stiffness in the limbs as a side effect of changing their diet from high acid to high alkaline. Massage can relieve this. Many of us are used to treating ourselves to a nice, relaxing massage in a beauty salon or spa as an occasional treat when we are on holiday but this is usually not effective enough to alleviate a persistent problem. I always recommend visiting an experienced masseur.

A particularly good penetrative treatment is with hot stones. These vary in size, and are usually made of basalt. They are placed in hot water until they reach a temperature where they are almost too hot to touch. The stones are smooth and round and retain heat well and have an excellent deep therapeutic effect. Passing the hot stones over the body makes the muscles loose and more responsive and easier to work on to release any stress. Combining the Holistic Detox with muscle-stretching exercises stimulates the cleansing process and keeps any muscular tension at bay.

Reflexology, which is a type of foot massage, is also an excellent complement to the Detox. In reflexology, the sole of the foot represents a map of the body, for example the toes correspond to the head, eyes and ears and the heel to the pelvic area. It has been practised for thousands of years by the Chinese and Egyptians and can work as a total body detox by helping to free stubbornly congested areas. It's particularly useful in the treatment of circulatory problems, digestive disorders, migraine, sinus and hormonal imbalances.

But just as when your GP prescribes a course of medication, it is important to approach any massage therapy as a course of treatments. It is not reasonable to expect your symptoms to disappear in one treatment, although they might. I recommend committing to four reflexology sessions for best results even though you may notice an improvement after just one. Similarly if you can commit to weekly massage sessions for a persistent problem you will achieve the best results. Talk to your therapist and see what he or she recommends.

It is important to drink a lot of water and avoid alcohol after a massage or reflexology session in order to flush out any toxins that may have been released, and rest afterwards. It is best to have a massage later in the day when you can go home afterwards and rest. You may experience discomfort the day after a deep massage. This is quite normal and is merely the result of the muscle reacting to being worked upon. It should only last a couple of days before the benefits start to show. If, however, the pain persists do not hesitate to visit your GP. The possible side effects of reflexology are a headache and mild nausea, resulting from the toxins that have been freed up from your congested organs working their way out of the body.

The ideal massage programme to complement the Holistic Detox is a deep-tissue or hot stone full body massage followed by a head massage, which has the effect of detoxing the skin so getting rid of spots and blemishes which may have been caused by sugar congestion, finishing up with some reflexology.

How to get the most out of massage

→ A good masseur will find any congested, stressed or tense muscles – you don't always have to tell him where they are, although it is advisable.

→ Let him know if he is working you too hard – you should not experience pain. Pain is a signal that something is going wrong. Some discomfort is to be expected, particularly in the neck and shoulder area but ask him to stop if you are in great discomfort.

→ Breathe through the massage. We expel many toxins through our breath and it is also important to keep the blood fed with a fresh oxygen supply.

→ There should be good communication between masseur and patient but don't distract your therapist by chatting to him constantly.

→ Many masseurs use oils during the treatment. Grapefruit oil is particularly good for cellulite and ylang ylang for facial skin problems.

→ Ask your masseur how long they have been working – make sure he has plenty of experience and is ITEC qualified.

MEDITATION

Meditation has been used for thousands of years in the East as a means of relaxing and enjoying quiet contemplation. The exercises are designed to allow the individual to create a mental environment divorced from the external influences and stresses of their physical and emotional life, and the demands of day-to-day living. The need to rely upon stimulants such as alcohol and recreational drugs in order to relax after a hectic day takes its toll on the body, whereas meditation enriches it while relaxing it at the same time.

MEDITATION EXERCISE

Close your eyes and focus on your breathing. Try to think of nothing else and you will begin to relax completely. Focus on your breath as you inhale and exhale and try to relax even more. You may find your mind wanders. It may think about things that have happened throughout the day or things you have to do, but try to keep focussed on your breath and encourage the screen within your mind's eye to be as blank as possible. Focus on a candle flame or create a mental picture of a place or painting or an environment like the seaside that automatically promotes a vision of calm. Keep your eyes closed. When you feel ready, become more aware of your surroundings and gradually open your eyes. Do this for 10–15 minutes as a way of relaxing at the end of each hectic day. By doing this you are encouraging your whole body to relax and your mind to detox.

The practice of meditation has been clinically shown to not only reduce cholesterol but to bring down high blood pressure as well as improving the general wellbeing of people suffering from conditions such as chronic stress, headaches, acidity, emotional vulnerability, skin irritations and insomnia. There are various types of meditation and in fact we meditate almost naturally every day without thinking about it, for example when we daydream, but to do it as a form of conscious concentration is more beneficial than drifting off in an uncontrolled manner.

Meditation is easily practised at home. It is best to sit in a warm room, either on the floor with your back against the wall or in a comfortable chair. The room should be dimly lit, perhaps by a candle. A bedroom is a good place. I like to precede my meditation with a hot shower. This helps me relax and rid my mind of the negative energies and thoughts I have absorbed throughout the day. It is important to be totally undisturbed during your meditation so make sure you are left alone by your family or housemates and switch the phone off. The process need only take 20–30 minutes. The first few times may take a little longer for you to feel relaxed but with practice you will be able to find a relaxed meditative state quite quickly. It is something I do at the end of every working day. Meditation creates a psychological divide between my work life and my personal life and refreshes me for whatever lies ahead.

There are other forms of meditation, such as transcendental meditation where you chant a mantra. Mantras are made up of Sanskrit words or sounds strung together to evoke a positive energy. The popular Sanskrit word 'om' for example, can be repeated aloud or silently to oneself, as a means to focus. In Hindu philosophy, meditation and mantras are designed to enable us to influence our environment, both internal and external.

Meditation can be taken even further by focussing on a chakra point – an energy centre in the body – through which powerful thought can influence organ function and hormonal balance and harmonise health. Detoxing the mind is a vital element in my Holistic Detox and mediation is a powerful tool to help us refresh, reboot and cleanse the mind – I urge you to try it.

Visualisation

Meditation is a wonderful foundation for visualisation exercises which have also been used for thousands of years to encourage positive influences in people's lives. Visualisation is a particularly powerful way of encouraging positive thought processes and patterns and eliminating negative thoughts about work, ourselves, our future or our relationships. Like meditation, it's something we actually do as part of everyday life: how many times have you rehearsed entire conversations to have with someone who has hurt or irritated you? You plan your speech over and over, getting more and more worked up; you visualise the entire scene in your mind. You even create the physical symptoms of anxiety – you get hot and bothered.

Visualisation exercises encourage us to use our mind's energies to help create a more positive future and look at things in a more optimistic and beneficial light. This can have a profoundly positive effect on our overall health, whether we are experiencing hormonal problems, circulation or digestion congestion, stress, insomnia or skin conditions.

VISUALISATION EXERCISE

After your meditation exercise, imagine there is a bright white light pouring through you from on high like a warm liquid penetrating the top of your head. It seeps right through and over you, onto your shoulders, down your arms, chest and back. It is a warm bright liquid that cleanses your body as it penetrates, moving down through your legs to your feet and forming roots deep beneath you stretching into the ground below. Imagine your body as this glowing, white form with a bright glowing future. Visualise what you would like to happen to you. See yourself going to a job interview and getting the job, imagine exactly how you want to look and feel in six months time, see yourself in a nurturing relationship with someone already in your life or someone new. Make the picture real, make it tangible so you can smell and taste it and feel exactly what it is like to be wherever you want to be.

Try to appreciate this image as something that is here and now. When you feel this, you can come out of this exercise by either covering the image with a protective white light or simply slowly coming back to an awareness of your immediate surroundings and open your eyes. Repeat this exercise as often as possible, daily if you can.

Many cancer patients are taught visualisation techniques as a means of using positive thoughts to irradiate the cancer or stem its progress. They visualise the cancer in their body as mud on their kitchen floor or dust on furniture or an untidy room. And as they visualise cleaning this dust or dirt, they are imagining that they are getting rid of the cancer in the bodies. I am not, of course, saying that visualisation exercises can cure cancer, but they can be very beneficial as part of a course of treatment and are a good way of empowering the individual rather than allowing them to surrender to silent resignation.

The adage that we can do anything we put our minds to has been proven many times, and the power of thought as a healer and cleanser is accepted by most conventional practitioners as well as alternative therapists. I practice visualisation exercises for ten minutes every morning before I get out of bed, and create a mental picture of all the positive things that are going to happen to me throughout the day. Then, after meditation in the evening, I may spend another ten minutes visualising positive events in the coming days. I recommend it to all my patients.

YOGA AND PILATES

Yoga is a Sanskrit word meaning union. First practised in India thousands of years ago, yoga is the ultimate holistic exercise incorporating mind, body and spirit. Many people are put off by yoga as they imagine it is just about trying to twist their limbs into impossible positions or standing on their head for hours on end. It really isn't like this at all. If we imagine our bodies as a bag of water which can only accumulate toxins then the physical practise of yoga works on moving that bag and the bits and pieces contained within it around so the toxins can be freed and released from the body. You don't need any special clothing or equipment to do yoga. It may seem a strange thing to say but breathing is quite fundamental to yoga and is something we should always think about when doing any kind of exercise or stretch. This is because we release a lot of our toxins through our breath which in turn stimulates our cardiovascular system.

A simple exercise for yoga novices is focussed breathing. Stand or sit and place your hands on your belly. Inhale and as you gently breathe out pull the belly away from your hands and continue to do this until you have no more breath. By doing this you are squeezing your intestines together and encouraging your diaphragm to pull up. Pulling your organs into a smaller space is like giving them an internal massage and helps problems such as constipation and bloating and can free blockages.

Relaxation is another vital component of yoga. This is a confusing concept as it is more than just a physical state: some people can be relaxed in a hectic situation and not relaxed quietly by themselves. Hanging off a doorframe is a great exercise to relieve stress and achieve relaxation. Stretch your shoulders and arms and neck into the stretch – try to hold this for about 30 seconds. Try to concentrate on the stretch as this will help you to relax mentally since you will not be thinking about anything else. It will take a while for your muscles to get the message to stretch, so hold it for as long as you can – a good stretch should last about two minutes. Do this as often as you can so you can build up to holding the stretch for longer periods of time. You may be aware of new sensations such as a rush of blood or warmth into a muscle. This is quite normal. The body will release tensions, as well as free any blockages

and toxins and because the mind has been focussing on the stretch it has not been worrying. The concentration on the physical allows a transfer of energy away from the past or future and into the present moment.

The presence of a teacher can be beneficial to ensure you do certain exercises correctly. Do try a class and see. There are lots of different types so try to persevere until you find one that suits you – yoga chooses you rather than you choosing yoga.

Yoga differs from other popular exercise techniques such as Pilates, which is also excellent for teaching core strength and flexibility. Some Pilates exercises are more about strengthening the stomach muscles for example, which in turn pulls up the pelvic floor. This is particularly good for posture and post-pregnancy. Yoga is a dynamic form of exercise and regards our internal organs as sponge-like substances, so the more they are twisted, stretched and extended, the more toxins can be got rid of. This dynamic movement helps to cleanse the digestive tract, which is what we are most concerned about during the Holistic Detox. Pilates is an excellent exercise to combine with yoga, though, because it lengthens limbs and is good for people wanting to recover their strength after an injury or to combat back pain. Yoga and Pilates concentrate on the entire body and cleanse it of stress and toxins through increasing suppleness and strength. But remember one size does not fit all, so listen to your body, pay attention to what you do and how you feel and in that way your body, mind and spirit are more likely to benefit.

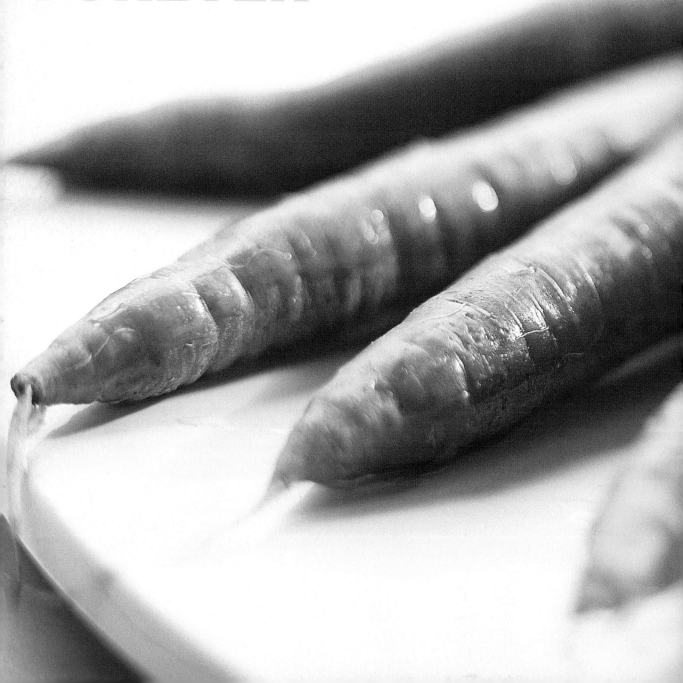

CHAPTER 9
HOLISTIC HEALTH FOREVER

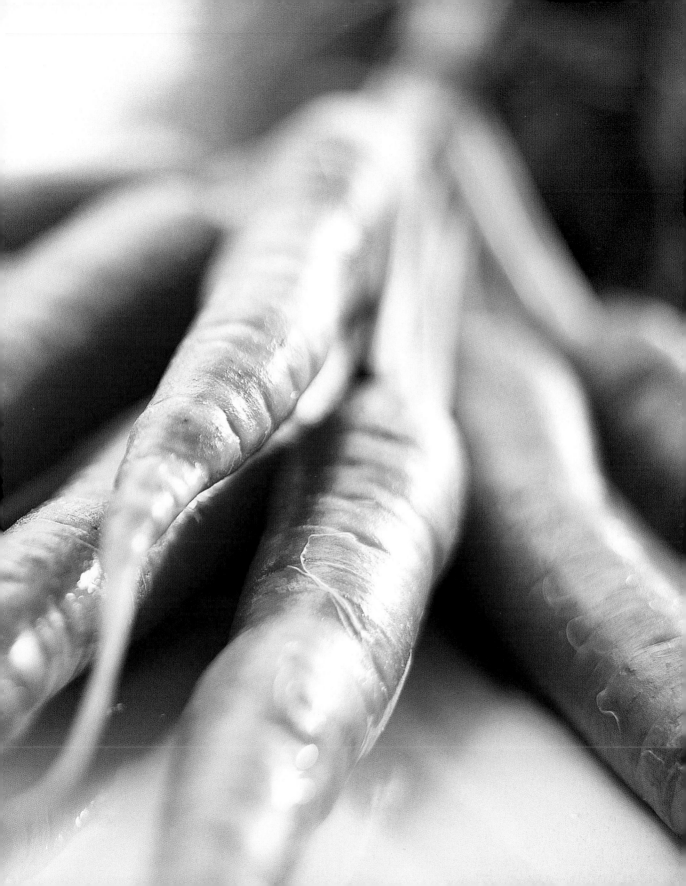

WELL, CONGRATULATIONS. HAVING COME THIS FAR, YOU WILL BE FEELING ALL THE BENEFITS OF MY HOLISTIC DETOX. YOU WILL BE LITERALLY GLOWING, YOUR EYES WILL BE SPARKLING, YOU WILL HAVE MORE ENERGY, YOUR HAIR WILL BE GLOSSIER AND YOUR SKIN CLEARER. YOU MAY ALSO HAVE BEEN ABLE TO STOP TAKING YOUR PRESCRIPTION MEDICINES AND WILL DEFINITELY BE FEELING YEARS YOUNGER. HOPEFULLY YOU WILL HAVE DISCOVERED A WHOLE HOST OF OTHER BENEFITS TOO, SUCH AS IMPROVED SLEEPING PATTERNS, A KEENER FOCUS ON YOUR JOB, BETTER CONCENTRATION AND MORE CONFIDENCE, ALL OF WHICH HELPS YOU TO COPE WITH AND JUGGLE ALL THE FACETS AND CHALLENGES IN YOUR LIFE. YOU MAY EVEN BE TIRING OF YOUR FRIENDS TELLING YOU HOW FABULOUS YOU LOOK AND HOW SLIM AND SEXY YOU ARE! IF YOU WEREN'T CONVINCED BEFORE YOU STARTED THE HOLISTIC DETOX, THEN YOU WILL BE NOW, OF THE RADICAL EFFECT SHIFTING AWAY FROM CERTAIN FOODS AND MOVING TOWARDS OTHERS CAN HAVE ON YOUR ENERGY LEVELS, GENERAL HEALTH AND WEIGHT.

Along the way you may have cheated and succumbed to an occasional bar of chocolate, packet of crisps or glass of wine. But you should have been pleasantly surprised by how little negative effect it had, providing you returned to the exciting new food regime I have prescribed for you.

Just because you have come to the end of the book does not mean you have come to the end of my Holistic Detox. In fact this is a new beginning. I have tried to give you all the tools you need to continue a healthy way of life, but now you are ready to go it alone, in the full knowledge that you can always refer to this book when you need to. In fact I recommend that you do just that every few months, if only to remind yourself of the foods on the acid/alkaline chart. I also advise that you revisit the 21- Day Detox plan every few months. You don't have to do it for the full three weeks, just a week should be sufficient to give your body the rest and cleanse it needs.

Here are my eight top tips to keep you eating healthily, feeling full of life and looking slim. This is the core of my Holistic Detox.

⤐ Meditate to start the day
⤐ Modify your shopping list to include fresh organic vegetables
⤐ Moderate your alcohol intake
⤐ Move around as much as possible and take plenty of exercise
⤐ Masticate your food eight times before you swallow
⤐ Mark your favourite recipes and experiment with them to stimulate your enjoyment of healthy new foods
⤐ Maintain a healthy balance of acid/alkaline forming foods
⤐ Make a commitment to your body to nurture it: supplying healthy food, sleep and exercise

Our quest for optimum wellbeing is so dependent on what we put in our mouths, as you now understand. And as you are feeling the benefits already, imagine how much more you can achieve if you commit to a truly healthy lifestyle. Enjoy!

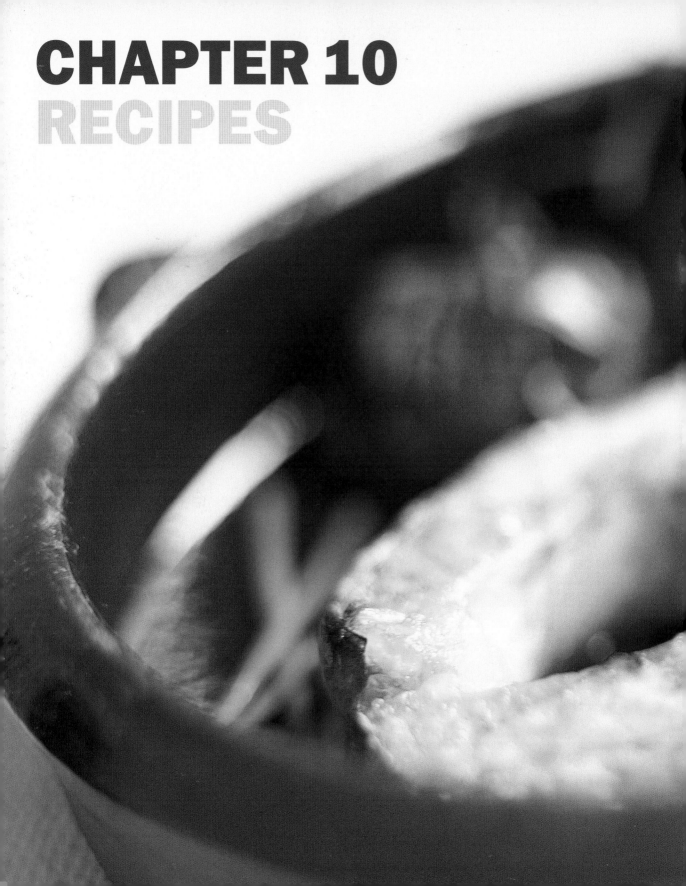

CHAPTER 10
RECIPES

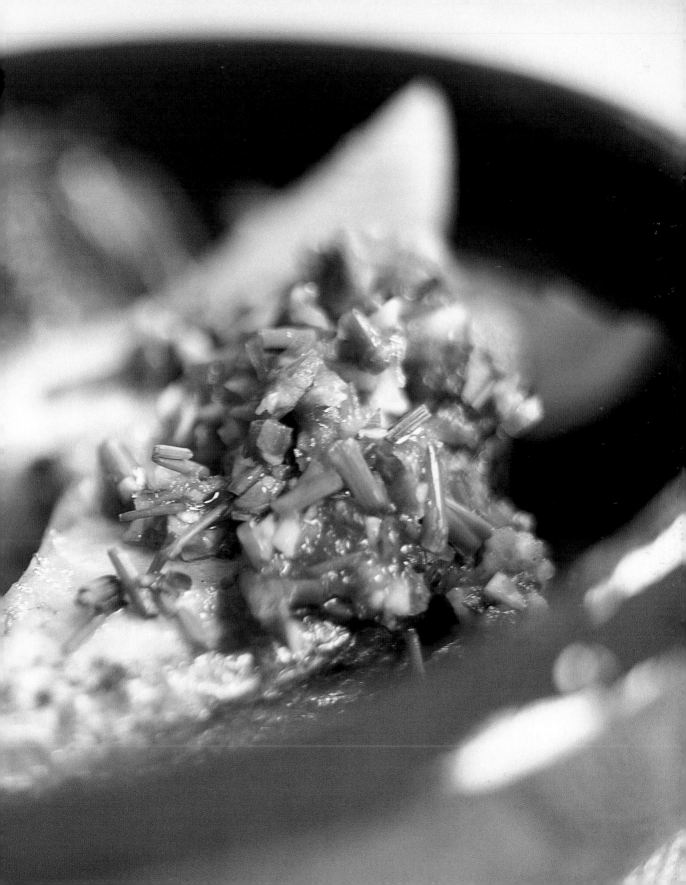

21-DAY DETOX

MOST OF THESE RECIPES ARE SPECIFICALLY DESIGNED FOR THE INITIAL 21-DAY DETOX, ALTHOUGH THEY CAN OF COURSE BE USED THROUGHOUT THE MAINTENANCE PHASE OF THE PROGRAMME AS WELL. THEY ARE INTENDED AS A STARTING POINT AND I WOULD ENCOURAGE YOU TO EXPERIMENT AS MUCH AS POSSIBLE – EATING SHOULD ALWAYS BE FUN!

SEVERAL OF THE RECIPES CALL FOR HOME MADE CHICKEN STOCK. THIS GIVES A FANTASTIC FLAVOUR AND IS EASY TO MAKE – SIMPLY BOIL UP ANY CHICKEN BONES OR, BETTER STILL A COMPLETE CARCASS, WITH A CARROT AND A BAY LEAF. SIMMER FOR HALF AN HOUR AND SKIM OFF ANY FAT. ALTERNATIVELY, YOU CAN USE A VEGETABLE BOUILLON CUBE. I RECOMMEND THAT IF YOU ARE MAKING UP STOCK, OR USING WATER TO COOK RICE OR MAKE SOUP, YOU USE FILTERED WATER WHERE POSSIBLE.

BREAKFAST

WHAT I CALL MY STANDARD BREAKFAST CONSISTS OF A NON-WHEAT GRAIN CEREAL WITH SOYA MILK. THIS KIND OF CEREAL, MADE WITH MILLET OR CORN AND WITH NO ADDED SUGAR, IS WIDELY AVAILABLE IN HEALTH FOOD SHOPS AND IS WORTH THE SEARCH. TRY SOME OF THE FOLLOWING ALTERNATIVES BY WAY OF VARIATION.

BREAKFAST PORRIDGE

2 SERVINGS
→ **2 CUPS WATER**
→ **1 CUP GLUTEN-FREE PORRIDGE**
→ **¼ TSP CINNAMON PLUS**
→ **A SPRINKLING TO SERVE**

In a medium saucepan, bring the cinnamon flavoured water to a boil. Pour in the porridge, reduce the heat to a simmer and cook for 30 seconds. Remove from heat, cover, and allow to stand for at least five minutes, until the liquid is absorbed. Top with a little more cinnamon and serve.

CHEESE AND CHIVE POLENTA

4 SERVINGS
→ **3 CUPS HOME MADE CHICKEN STOCK**
→ **1 AND ¼ CUPS CORNMEAL**
→ **1 TBSP CHIVES, FINELY CHOPPED**
→ **1 TBSP PARSLEY, FINELY CHOPPED**
→ **2 TBSP OLIVE OIL**
→ **50G/2 OZ SOYA CHEESE OR
   BUFFALO MOZZARELLA, CRUMBLED**

Bring the stock to the boil in a large saucepan. Gradually whisk in the cornmeal. Lower the heat and cook, stirring constantly, until the mixture starts to thicken. Immediately whisk in the chives, parsley, cheese, and two tablespoons of olive oil. When the cornmeal has thickened, dot with a little olive oil. You can serve the polenta as is or, for a special treat, sauté in olive oil.

EGGS FLORENTINE

4 SERVINGS
→ **1 CUP BROWN RICE**
→ **4–8 EGGS**
→ **1 SMALL WHITE ONION,**
→ **FINELY CHOPPED**
→ **4 COOKED ARTICHOKE BASES,
   (BUY THE ONES IN WATER, NOT OIL)**
→ **1 TBSP OLIVE OIL**
→ **1 LARGE BUNCH SPINACH,
   ROUGHLY CHOPPED**
→ **PINCH OF NUTMEG**
→ **DASH OF PAPRIKA**

Cook the rice. Sauté the onion in olive oil until translucent, add the spinach and cook until soft, no more than three minutes. Add the nutmeg and stir through. Set aside and keep warm. Poach the eggs in about an inch of simmering water for three to five minutes. Put the artichoke bottoms on hot plates then spread with the spinach mixture. Top each one with one or two poached eggs. Drizzle over a little extra olive oil and a dash of paprika. Serve with the hot rice.

LUNCH

TRY TO GET INTO THE HABIT OF PREPARING SOME OF THESE LUNCH DISHES IN ADVANCE SO THAT YOU CAN TAKE THEM INTO WORK OR HAVE THEM EASILY AVAILABLE IF YOU'RE ON THE GO. SOME OF THEM CALL FOR HOMEMADE MAYONNAISE, WHICH IS PREFERABLE TO THE SHOP-BOUGHT VARIETY AS IT DOESN'T CONTAIN VINEGAR. THIS IS SURPRISINGLY EASY TO MAKE. GENTLY COMBINE FOUR EGG YOLKS WITH A TABLESPOON OF LEMON JUICE IN A FOOD PROCESSOR. KEEP THE MOTOR RUNNING VERY SLOWLY AS YOU GRADUALLY ADD A QUARTER OF A CUP OF OLIVE OIL BY POURING IN A THIN STREAM. TURN OFF WHEN THE OIL IS ALL ADDED AND ADD A LITTLE MORE LEMON JUICE, TO TASTE. SET ASIDE AND REFRIGERATE UNTIL REQUIRED. IT WILL LAST FOR UP TO A MONTH IF KEPT CHILLED IN A SEALED CONTAINER. ASIDE FROM SANDWICHES AND SOUPS, SOME OF THE BEST LUNCH DISHES ARE ENTIRELY COMPOSED OF VEGETABLES. TRY STEAMING VEGETABLES SUCH AS ASPARAGUS, BROCCOLI OR SNAP PEAS AND SEASONING WITH OLIVE OIL AND FRESH HERBS. GET INVENTIVE AND EXPERIMENT WITH DIFFERENT COMBINATIONS.

CHICKEN SALAD SANDWICH

6 SERVINGS
- 1 ROASTED CHICKEN, SKINNED AND CHOPPED
- ¾ CUP HOMEMADE MAYONNAISE
- 3 STICKS CELERY, CHOPPED
- RICE CAKES OR TORTILLAS

Strip as much meat from the chicken as you can. Reserve the carcass for stock. Toss all ingredients in a bowl and spread on rice cakes or wrap up in tortillas.

BEAN SOUP

4 SERVINGS
- 4 CUPS CHICKEN STOCK
- 3 CUPS WHITE BEANS, COOKED OVERNIGHT OR TINNED
- 1 LARGE CARROT, SLICED
- 1 SMALL ONION, FINELY CHOPPED
- 2 TBSP LEMON JUICE

Combine stock, carrots, onion, and lemon juice in a saucepan. Simmer, covered, until carrots are just tender. Stir in beans. Heat thoroughly.

SPECIAL CHICKEN SOUP

4 SERVINGS
- → **6 CUPS CHICKEN STOCK**
- → **1KG/2 LBS BONED CHICKEN MEAT, TRIMMED AND FINELY CHOPPED**
- → **⅓ CUP COOKED NON-WHEAT PASTA**
- → **JUICE OF 1 LEMON OR LIME**
- → **2 EGGS**
- → **2 TBSP CORIANDER, FINELY CHOPPED**

Heat stock and add chicken pieces. Simmer until meat is cooked: about five minutes. Add the pasta, bring to a simmer and remove from heat. Squeeze three tablespoons of the lime or lemon juice into a bowl, add the eggs and whisk together. Gradually add two cups of the broth to the egg mixture, whisking constantly, then slowly whisk the eggs into the soup mixture. Return to low heat until soup starts to steam. Add coriander and serve at once.

CARROT SOUP

4 SERVINGS
- → **1 MEDIUM ONION, SLICED VERY THIN**
- → **2 TBSP OLIVE OIL**
- → **8 MEDIUM CARROTS, SLICED**
- → **2 CUPS CHICKEN STOCK**
- → **1 TBSP FRESH GINGER, MINCED**
- → **1 TBSP FRESH THYME LEAVES**

In a large saucepan, cook the onion in the olive oil until translucent. Add the carrots and stock and simmer, Purée the carrot mixture in batches in a food processor or blender. Transfer the purée to the saucepan, add the ginger and thyme and simmer, stirring, for 10 minutes. Serve at once.

DINNER

THESE DISHES ARE A LITTLE MORE SUBSTANTIAL
THAN THE LIGHT LUNCH DISHES BUT THEY CAN,
OF COURSE, ALSO BE EATEN AT LUNCHTIME;
SIMPLY MAKE THEM IN ADVANCE AND TAKE
THEM INTO WORK.

BRUSSELS SPROUTS AND CARROTS

6 SERVINGS
- → 500G/1LB BRUSSELS SPROUTS, TRIMMED AND HALVED
- → 500G/1LB CARROTS, PEELED AND SLICED
- → 1 TSP CARAWAY SEEDS
- → 1 GARLIC CLOVE, FINELY CHOPPED
- → GRATED PEEL OF ONE LEMON
- → 2 TBSP LEMON JUICE
- → 2 TBSP OLIVE OIL

In a large saucepan, cook the Brussels sprouts and carrots in one inch of boiling water until tender, about 10–15 minutes. Drain well and set vegetables aside. In the same pan, add the caraway seeds, garlic, lemon peel, and lemon juice to the olive oil and cook gently for one minute. Add the cooked vegetables and heat through.

PARSNIP AND BEET FRY

2 SERVINGS

→ **1 MEDIUM BEET, UNPEELED**
→ **1 MEDIUM PARSNIP, PEELED
AND GRATED**
→ **3 TBSP OLIVE OIL**
→ **1 TBSP SHALLOT, FINELY CHOPPED**
→ **1/4 TSP DRIED THYME, CRUMBLED**
→ **FRESH THYME SPRIGS**

Preheat oven to 180°C/350°F. Place the beet in a small baking pan and bake until tender, about one hour. Remove from oven and allow to cool, then grate and combine with the parsnip and crumbled thyme. Lightly sauté the shallot in a tablespoon of olive oil then add the beet and parsnip mixture and cook for about three minutes. Add the remaining two tablespoons of oil and cook over a low heat, stirring occasionally, for 10 minutes. Sprinkle with thyme sprigs and serve.

BRUSSELS SPROUTS WITH PECAN BUTTER

6 SERVINGS

→ **3/4 CUP PECAN NUTS,
FINELY CHOPPED**
→ **2 TBSPS OLIVE OIL**
→ **1 KG/2 LBS BRUSSELS SPROUTS,
TRIMMED**
→ **4 TBSP OLIVE OIL**

Cook the pecans over low heat in the olive oil until lightly browned, about 15 minutes. Steam the Brussels sprouts until tender and add to the pecan butter. Heat through, stirring occasionally.

SPICY WILD RICE

6 SERVINGS
→ **2 TBSP OLIVE OIL**
→ **1 CARROT, DICED**
→ **1 STICK CELERY, DICED**
→ **1 LEEK, WASHED AND SLICED**
→ **2 CUPS BROWN RICE**
→ **4 CUPS CHICKEN STOCK, PLUS EXTRA AS REQUIRED**
→ **1 TSP CUMIN**
→ **1 TSP CINNAMON**

Gently heat the olive oil and add the carrot, celery, and leek. Cook, stirring occasionally, for about one minute. Stir in the rice and the spices and add the chicken stock. Cover, and cook slowly until rice is done, about one hour and 15 minutes. Add extra chicken stock as needed.

LENTIL PILAF

6 SERVINGS
→ **2 TBSP OLIVE OIL**
→ **1 BUNCH SPRING ONIONS, CHOPPED**
→ **2 GARLIC CLOVES, FINELY CHOPPED**
→ **1 CUP LENTILS, RINSED**
→ **1/2 CUP BROWN RICE, RINSED**
→ **1/4 CUP WILD RICE, RINSED**
→ **2 TBSP FLAKED ALMONDS**
→ **1/2 TSP DRIED THYME**
→ **2 1/2 CUPS CHICKEN STOCK**

In a large saucepan, sauté the onions, garlic, lentils, and both types of rice in the olive oil until the onion is tender, about four minutes. Add the almonds, thyme, and chicken stock and bring to a boil. Reduce heat and simmer, covered, for about 30 minutes or until the liquid is absorbed.

RED BEANS AND RICE

6 SERVINGS

BEANS:
- 500G/1LB DRIED RED KIDNEY BEANS
- 2 TBSP OLIVE OIL
- 4 GARLIC CLOVES, FINELY CHOPPED
- 2 CUPS ONION, CHOPPED
- 4 CUPS CHICKEN STOCK
- 2 BAY LEAVES

RICE:
- 2 TBSP OLIVE OIL
- 1 SMALL ONION, CHOPPED
- 2 CUPS LONG-GRAIN RICE, FRESHLY COOKED

Beans: Place beans in a bowl, cover with water, and soak for 24 hours. Drain and set aside. In a large saucepan, sauté the onion in olive oil over low heat until it's golden brown, about 15 minutes. Add the garlic and sauté for another three minutes. Add the beans and chicken stock, bring to a boil and then simmer, covered, for about two hours taking care not to let the beans stick. Add the bay leaves and continue to simmer, covered, until the beans are tender: about another hour. Transfer to a bowl and keep warm.

Rice: Sauté the onion in the olive oil until tender, about 10 minutes. Add the rice and heat through. Serve rice and beans together.

MARINATED BASS WITH CORIANDER

4 SERVINGS
- → 4, 6OZ BASS (OR HALIBUT OR ANY OTHER WHITE FISH) FILLETS
- → JUICE OF 2 LIMES
- → 2 TBSP OLIVE OIL
- → 1 GARLIC CLOVE, FINELY CHOPPED
- → 3 TBSP FRESH CORIANDER, CHOPPED
- → LIME WEDGES

Place the fish in a shallow dish and pour the lime juice over them. Marinate in the fridge for at least 30 minutes. Very gently, cook the garlic in the olive oil for about 30 seconds. Add the coriander and cook until heated through, about 1 minute. On a medium-hot grill, cook the fish for about 8–10 minutes, depending on the thickness of the fillets, basting frequently with the coriander butter. Serve garnished with lime wedges.

CARPACCIO OF SALMON WITH LIME

4 SERVINGS
- → 500G/1LB SALMON FILLETS
- → 2 SHALLOTS, FINELY CHOPPED
- → 4 TBSP OLIVE OIL
- → JUICE OF 1/2 LIME
- → PEEL OF ONE LIME, GRATED

Put four ovenproof plates in a preheated oven to warm, then cut the salmon into paper-thin slices and set aside. Sauté the shallots in olive oil until slightly brown. Squeeze in the lime juice and sprinkle in the peel, stirring as you add them. When the mixture sizzles, coat each warmed plate with half a tablespoon of it and immediately add fish. Pour the remaining lime oil over the salmon and serve immediately.

GRILLED MARINATED CHICKEN BREASTS

4 SERVINGS
→ ¾ CUP LEMON JUICE
→ ¾ CUP VEGETABLE OIL
→ ½ SMALL ONION, FINELY CHOPPED
→ 1½ TSP DRIED THYME
→ 8 CHICKEN BREASTS, BONED AND SKINNED
→ FRESH THYME FOR GARNISHING

In a medium bowl, mix together the lemon juice, oil, onion, and thyme. With a sharp knife, make small cuts in each chicken breast. Pour one third of the marinade into a shallow glass bowl or baking dish. Add half the chicken and cover with one third of the marinade. Layer the remaining chicken on top and add the remaining marinade. Allow to stand in the refrigerator for three hours, turning occasionally. Remove from the refrigerator for an hour to bring to room temperature. Grill the chicken for about three minutes on each side, taking care not to overcook. Garnish with fresh thyme.

CHICKEN AND FRESH HERB PESTO

4 SERVINGS
- **4 SPRING ONIONS, FINELY CHOPPED**
- **2 TBSP WALNUT PIECES OR PINE NUTS**
- **1–1/2 TSP GRATED LEMON PEEL**
- **4 LARGE GARLIC CLOVES**
- **2 TBSP FRESH ITALIAN PARSLEY LEAVES**
- **2 TBSP FRESH TARRAGON OR BASIL LEAVES**
- **1/2 CUP OLIVE OIL**
- **4 WHOLE CHICKEN LEGS**

Preheat the oven to 230°/450°F. Mix the first six ingredients in a food processor. While the machine is running, add oil slowly until the mixture is a coarse paste. Grease a baking dish with a little olive oil for the chicken pieces and spread them with pesto. Bake until tender, about 40 minutes, basting once with the pesto mixture.

BAKED CHICKEN WITH ROOT VEGETABLES

4 SERVINGS
- → **2 LARGE CARROTS, PEELED AND CUT INTO 1 INCH PIECES**
- → **2 PARSNIPS, PEELED AND CUT INTO 1 INCH PIECES**
- → **1 MEDIUM ONION, QUARTERED**
- → **1 RUTABAGA, PEELED AND CUT INTO 1 INCH PIECES**
- → **2 TBSP PLUS 2 TSP OLIVE OIL**
- → **1 TSP SAGE**
- → **1 TSP DRIED ROSEMARY**
- → **4 CHICKEN DRUMSTICKS AND 4 THIGH PIECES**
- → **2 GARLIC CLOVES, CRUSHED**

Preheat the oven to 190°C/375°F. Put the carrots, parsnips, rutabaga, and onion in a baking pan. Add two tablespoons of oil, 1/2 teaspoon of sage, and 1/2 teaspoon rosemary and stir through. Bake, covered, for 30 minutes. Meanwhile, rub the chicken with garlic, then with the remaining oil, sage, and rosemary. Add the chicken to the vegetables. Cook for an additional hour, stirring the vegetables occasionally.

ROAST CHICKEN WITH GARLIC

4 SERVINGS
- → **1 LARGE CHICKEN**
- → **10 LARGE GARLIC CLOVES**
- → **1 TBSP DRIED OREGANO**
- → **2 TBSP OLIVE OIL**
- → **3 TBSP CHICKEN STOCK**

Preheat oven to 230°C/450°F. Rinse chicken and pat dry. Place breast side up on a foil lined roasting pan. Split eight garlic cloves and add, with 1/2 tablespoon of oregano, to chicken cavity. Mince the remaining garlic and mix with the remaining oregano, oil, and the stock. Carefully separate skin from breast area of chicken and spoon half of garlic mixture under skin. Smear the remaining garlic mixture over surface of chicken. Roast until the juices from the thigh have turned from rosy to clear, allow to rest for 10 minutes, then carve and serve.

LEMON CHICKEN WITH CAPERS

4 SERVINGS
→ 1/4 CUP PINE NUTS
→ 4 SKINLESS CHICKEN BREASTS, BONED
→ 1 TBSP OLIVE OIL
→ 1/2 CUP CHICKEN STOCK
→ 1 1/2 TBSP FRESH LEMON JUICE
→ 1 TBSP CAPERS

Toast the pine nuts in an oven preheated to 200°C/400°F. It won't take long, just a couple of minutes, so keep an eye on them. Set aside to cool. Gently pound the chicken breasts between sheets of waxed paper until flattened. In a large frying pan, heat the oil over a moderately high heat until almost smoking. Add the breasts and cook until golden brown, about five minutes. Turn over and cook until white throughout but still moist, about an additional three minutes. Arrange the chicken on a large platter and cover with foil to keep warm. Pour off any fat from the pan, add the chicken stock and bring to a boil, scraping up any brown bits from the bottom of the pan. Cook over a high heat until reduced by half, about three minutes. Add the lemon juice and capers, remove from heat and add any accumulated juices from the platter of chicken. Pour sauce over the chicken and sprinkle with pine nuts.

TURKEY THIGHS WITH VEGETABLE SAUCE

4 SERVINGS
- 8 TURKEY THIGHS, SKINNED
- 1–1/2 TSP OREGANO
- 1–1/2 CUPS CHICKEN STOCK
- 1–1/2 TBSP OLIVE OIL
- 1 ONION, SLICED
- 1 MEDIUM MARROW, SLICED
- 1 BUNCH RADISH, CUT INTO HALVES
- JUICE OF 1 LEMON
- 2 TBSP FRESH BASIL, CHOPPED

Rub the turkey thighs lightly with oil, sprinkle with oregano and place in a baking dish. Cover with one cup of stock and bake at 160°C/325°F for an hour, basting occasionally. Heat the olive oil in a frying pan and sauté the onion until tender. Stir in the marrow and radish and sauté for three minutes. Add the remaining stock and lemon juice and simmer until vegetables are tender-crisp. Add the basil and stir until heated through. Serve with vegetables on the side.

CHICKEN CURRY

4 SERVINGS

→ **8 CHICKEN THIGHS, SKINNED**
→ **1 CUP SOYA YOGURT**
→ **1 TSP GROUND GINGER**
→ **1/2 TSP GROUND TURMERIC**
→ **1 TSP GARLIC, MINCED**
→ **1 CUP VEGETABLE OIL**
→ **2 ONIONS, FINELY CHOPPED**
→ **1 TBSP GROUND CORIANDER**
→ **1 TBSP GROUND CUMIN**
→ **1 TBSP GROUND ALMONDS**
→ **1/2 CUP SHREDDED COCONUT**
→ **1/4 TSP GROUND NUTMEG**
→ **1/4 TSP GROUND MACE**
→ **1/2 TSP GROUND CINNAMON**
→ **1/2 TSP GROUND CLOVES**
→ **1 TBSP GROUND CARDAMOM**
→ **1 CUP WARM WATER**
→ **1 CUP SOYA MILK**
→ **1/4 TSP SAFFRON**
→ **1/2 CUP CHOPPED CORIANDER LEAVES**
→ **1/4 CUP LEMON JUICE**

Pierce the chicken thighs with a fork then mix together the yogurt, ginger, turmeric, and garlic. Rub over the chicken and marinate in the refrigerator for two hours. Heat the oil in a large frying pan and sauté the onions until golden. Reserving the oil, remove the onions and set aside to cool. In the same pan, cook the coriander, cumin, almonds, coconut, nutmeg, and mace over a medium-low heat for three minutes, stirring constantly. Add the onions, transfer the mixture to a blender and grind to a fine paste. Add the cinnamon, cloves, and cardamom and stir through. Cook the chicken pieces gently in the same frying pan, turning until done, about 20–25 minutes. Pour the spice paste over the chicken and top with any leftover yogurt marinade. Add the warm water and simmer until the chicken is tender. In a small saucepan, warm the soya milk and add the saffron. When heated through, add it gradually to the chicken, stirring slowly, cooking for two more minutes. Before serving, sprinkle the chicken with the coriander and lemon juice. Serve with rice.

MAINTENANCE

DO BEAR IN MIND THAT THESE RECIPES ARE VERY MUCH SUGGESTIONS. IT IS IMPORTANT TO RE-INTRODUCE ALL FOODS GRADUALLY, USING YOUR FOOD DIARY TO RECORD ANY PROBLEMS AND ACCORDING TO YOUR OWN AYURVEDIC METABOLIC TYPE. OF COURSE, AS YOU BROADEN THE RANGE OF FOODS YOU'RE EATING, YOU WILL BE ABLE TO ADAPT FAVOURITE RECIPES FROM ELSEWHERE. THESE ARE A FEW IDEAS TO GET YOU STARTED.

LUNCH
TUNA SALAD SANDWICH

2 SERVINGS
→ 1 SMALL TIN TUNA (IN OIL, NOT BRINE)
→ 1 SMALL RED ONION, DICED
→ ¼ CUP HOMEMADE MAYONNAISE
→ 6 RICE CAKES
→ BUTTER (A LITTLE, FOR SPREADING)
→ ¼ CUP FRESH PARSLEY, CHOPPED

Combine tuna, mayonnaise, and onion and mix well. Butter the rice cakes, top with the tuna mixture and garnish with parsley. You can add one or more of the following ingredients to vary your sandwich: chopped coriander or basil, chopped celery, curry powder, lemon juice, tomato slices.

SHRIMP AND CORN SALAD

4 SERVINGS
→ 2 CUPS SWEETCORN
→ 250G/½ LB SMALL COOKED SHRIMP
→ ½ CUP HOMEMADE MAYONNAISE
→ 2 STICKS CELERY, CHOPPED
→ 3 SPRING ONIONS, CHOPPED
→ ¼ TSP CURRY POWDER

Combine all the ingredients and refrigerate for at least one hour before serving.

CALIFORNIA SALAD

4 SERVINGS

→ 500G/1 LB RIPE TOMATOES,
  CUT INTO WEDGES
→ 2 TBSP FRESH BASIL LEAVES
→ 250G/1/2 LB YELLOW CHERRY
  TOMATOES
→ 1 SMALL RED ONION, CHOPPED
→ 1/4 CUP OLIVE OIL
→ 2 TBSP LEMON JUICE

In a large bowl, combine the tomatoes, basil, onion, and oil. Toss well, add lemon juice and toss again.

LENTIL SOUP

4 SERVINGS

→ 1 CUP RED OR GREEN LENTILS
→ 3 CUPS WATER
→ 1 CARROT, DICED
→ 1 SMALL ONION, CHOPPED
→ 1 BAY LEAF
→ 1/2 TSP THYME
→ 500G/1 LB TOMATOES, CHOPPED
  OR ONE LARGE CAN TOMATOES
→ 2 TBSP BUTTER

Rinse lentils thoroughly. Place in a saucepan with water, carrot, onion, bay leaf, and thyme. Bring to a boil over medium heat, cover and simmer over a low heat for 45 minutes. Add butter and tomatoes. Heat through and serve.

TOMATO AND GARLIC SOUP

4 SERVINGS

→ 4 MEDIUM GARLIC CLOVES, MINCED
→ 2 TBSP OLIVE OIL
→ 1 KG/2 LBS ITALIAN PLUM
   TOMATOES, PEELED, SEEDED
   AND CHOPPED
→ 6 CUPS CHICKEN STOCK
→ FRESH BASIL LEAVES, TORN

In a large saucepan, sauté the garlic in the olive oil over a low heat. Add the tomatoes and cook gently, uncovered, for about 10 minutes, stirring frequently. Add the chicken stock and simmer for 20 minutes. Stir in the basil and serve hot or chilled, adding basil as garnish.

FRENCH ONION SOUP

2 SERVINGS

→ 50G/2 OZ ONION, FINELY CHOPPED
→ 1 TBSP OLIVE OIL
→ 25G/1 OZ CARROT, CHOPPED
→ 1 CUP ORGANIC BROWN RICE
→ 25G/1 OZ TOMATO, CHOPPED
→ 3 CUPS FILTERED WATER
→ LEMON JUICE AND BLACK PEPPER
   FOR SEASONING

Sauté the onion in the olive oil until translucent. Cook the rice with the tomato and carrot in three cups of filtered water until very tender. Add the onion and some more water and simmer hard for a further five minutes. Add lemon juice and pepper to taste.

MIXED VEGETABLE SOUP

2 SERVINGS

→ **1 OZ/25G PEAS**
→ **2 OZS/50G SPINACH,
  ROUGHLY CHOPPED**
→ **2 OZS/50G CABBAGE,
  FINELY CHOPPED**
→ **2 OZS/50G BEETROOT,
  FINELY CHOPPED**
→ **2 OZS/50G CUCUMBER, DICED**
→ **2 OZS/50G TOMATO, DICED**
→ **3 CUPS CHICKEN STOCK**
→ **LEMON JUICE AND BLACK PEPPER
  FOR SEASONING**

Steam the chopped vegetables and then whiz to a pulp in a blender. Add to the stock or water with a pinch of salt and simmer for 5–10 minutes. Adjust seasoning to taste and serve immediately.

DINNER
CORIANDER RICE

2 SERVINGS
- → 1 TBSP CORIANDER LEAVES
- → 3 CLOVES GARLIC
- → 2 GREEN CHILLIES, SEEDED
- → 2 TBSP OLIVE OIL
- → 25G/1 OZ CARROT
- → 25G/1 OZ BUTTER BEANS
- → 100G/4 OZ ORGANIC BASMATI RICE
- → 2 CUPS FILTERED WATER

Whizz the green chillies, coriander and garlic in a blender to make a paste. Heat the oil in a large saucepan and sauté the carrot for five minutes. Add the beans, paste and rice and sauté for a further couple of minutes. Add three cups of water and leave to simmer gently until the rice is cooked, adding more water as required.

GARLIC BROCCOLI WITH PENNE

4 SERVINGS
- → 225G/1/2 LB GLUTEN-FREE PASTA
- → 500G/1 LB BROCCOLI, CHOPPED INTO SMALL PIECES
- → 4 GARLIC CLOVES, MINCED
- → 1 TBSP OLIVE OIL
- → BLACK PEPPER TO SEASON
- → BUFFALO MOZZARELLA TO GARNISH

Boil the pasta until *al dente*. Meanwhile, sauté the broccoli and garlic in the olive oil over a medium heat until the broccoli turns bright green. Toss with the pasta and season and garnish according to taste. Serve immediately.

VEGETABLE PILAF

4 SERVINGS
- 125G/5 OZ ORGANIC BASMATI RICE
- 1 TBSP SUNFLOWER OIL
- 1 TSP CUMIN SEEDS
- 3 OR 4 CURRY LEAVES
- 3 GREEN CHILLIES, MINCED
- 2 CLOVES GARLIC, MINCED
- 2 INCH PIECE GINGER, MINCED
- 1 LARGE ONION, FINELY CHOPPED
- 25G/ 1 OZ PEAS
- 25G/1 OZ CARROTS, FINELY CHOPPED
- 25G/1 OZ BUTTER BEANS
- 1/2 TSP TURMERIC POWDER
- 2 CUPS FILTERED WATER
- LEMON JUICE AND BLACK PEPPER FOR SEASONING

Wash and soak the rice and set to one side. Heat the oil in a large saucepan and when slightly smoking, add the cumin seeds, curry leaves, green chillies and the garlic and ginger. Sauté gently for a couple of minutes and then add the onions and cook until translucent. Add the vegetables and beans and sauté for a further three minutes, then add the turmeric powder and mix through. Add the rice and two cups of water and keep adding more as required. Serve hot when the rice is cooked and all the water has been absorbed. This is a really adaptable recipe; you can vary the vegetables and beans according to your taste.

CHICKEN PROVENÇAL

4 SERVINGS
- 4 CHICKEN BREASTS, SKINNED AND BONED
- 1 TBSP OLIVE OIL
- 120G/4 OZ SOYA CHEESE OR BUFFALO MOZZARELLA
- 4 SMALL TOMATOES, SLICED
- 1 TBSP CHOPPED FRESH ROSEMARY
- 1/2 CUP CHICKEN STOCK

Place the chicken breasts between sheets of waxed paper and gently pound until flattened. Over a medium-high heat, heat the oil in a large frying pan and sauté the chicken breasts until golden on both sides. Arrange alternating slices of cheese and tomato on each breast and sprinkle with rosemary. Pour the stock over the chicken and cover. Lower heat and cook for about three minutes, until cheese and tomato are cooked through. Remove the chicken to a warm platter and high boil sauce rapidly down, over a high heat. Pour sauce over chicken.

SWORDFISH WITH MINT AND LEMON BUTTER

4 SERVINGS
→ 50G/2 OZ UNSALTED BUTTER,
  AT ROOM TEMPERATURE
→ 4 TSP FRESH MINT, FINELY CHOPPED
→ 1 TSP LEMON PEEL, GRATED
→ 4, 6OZ SWORDFISH STEAKS
→ 1/4 CUP OLIVE OIL
→ FRESH MINT LEAVES

Mix the butter, chopped mint and lemon peel in a small bowl. Cover and refrigerate. Put the fish in a shallow baking dish and drizzle with oil. Grill or broil fish until pink inside, about four minutes a side. Transfer the fish to plates and top with a thick slice of mint and lemon butter. Garnish with mint leaves.

BRAISED ROOT VEGETABLES

6 SERVINGS
→ 25G/1 OZ BUTTER
→ 4 GARLIC CLOVES, MINCED
→ 1 ONION, SLICED
→ 250G/1/2 LB CARROTS,
  PEELED AND SLICED
→ 500G/1 LB SWEET POTATOES,
  PEELED AND SLICED
→ 250G/1/2 LB PARSNIPS,
  PEELED AND SLICED
→ 2 TBSP PARSLEY, CHOPPED

Melt half the butter in a large frying pan, add the garlic and onion and cook until translucent. Add carrots, sweet potatoes, parsnips, and water to cover. Bring to a boil and then simmer, covered, until vegetables are just tender but not mushy: about 20 minutes. Remove lid and bring to a rapid boil. When liquid has evaporated, add remaining butter in pieces, stirring so vegetables are fully coated, and sprinkle with parsley.

GRILLED SALMON WITH TOMATOES AND HERBS

4 SERVINGS

→ 3 TOMATOES, PEELED, SEEDED, AND CHOPPED
→ 1/2 CUP OLIVE OIL
→ 3 TBSP LEMON JUICE
→ 3 GARLIC CLOVES, MINCED
→ 2 TBSP CHERVIL, CHOPPED
→ 2 TBSP CHIVES, CHOPPED
→ 2 TBSP TARRAGON, CHOPPED
→ 4 SALMON (OR TUNA) STEAKS

Lightly fry the tomatoes and garlic in the olive oil, add the lemon juice and garlic. Set aside for two hours then add all the herbs, mixing well. Grill the fish, turning once, until charred on the outside, about three to four minutes on each side. Transfer the fish to a large platter and top with the tomato sauce.

CHICKEN AND SQUASH WITH HERB BUTTER

4 SERVINGS

→ 50G/2 OZ BUTTER, AT ROOM TEMPERATURE
→ 2 GARLIC CLOVES, MINCED
→ 2 TBSP FRESH BASIL, TARRAGON, OR PARSLEY, CHOPPED
→ 4 WHOLE CHICKEN LEGS
→ 2 YELLOW SQUASH, THINLY SLICED
→ 2 COURGETTES, THINLY SLICED

Mix the butter, garlic, and herbs together. Preheat the oven to 220°C/425°F. Dot a tablespoon of the herb butter under the skin of each chicken leg and bake in the oven for 35 minutes. Just before the chicken is done, heat the rest of the herb butter in a large pan. Add the squash and courgettes and sauté until tender, a few minutes at most. Serve the chicken surrounded by the squash.

DRINKS
CLEANSING DRINK

PART 1:
→ 1 HEAPED TSP OF PSYLLIUM HUSKS
→ $1/2$ TSP OF BENTONITE CLAY
→ 1 CUP FILTERED OR SPRING WATER
→ $1/4$ CUP ORGANIC APPLE JUICE

First, combine the husks and clay, then add the water and juice and drink immediately.

PART 2:
→ 1 TSP RAW HONEY
→ 1 TSP CIDER VINEGAR
→ 1 CUP FILTERED WATER

Combine all the ingredients and drink after the first part of the cleansing drink, first thing in the morning once into the Maintenance phase of the Holistic Detox unless you are suffering from candida. At other times of the day (but not at the same time), supplement these cleansing drinks with raw vegetable juices and fruit juices. Try not to drink vegetable juices and fruit juices within 1–2 hours of each other.

DIRECTORY

FOOD SUPPLIERS AND PRODUCERS

The Soil Association
The UK's leading campaigning
and certification organisation
for organic food and farming.
Bristol House, 40–56 Victoria Street
Bristol BS1 6BY
T: 0117 314 5000
E: info@soilassociation.org
Website: www.soilassociation.org

Soil Association Scotland
18 Liberton Brae, Tower Mains
Edinburgh, EH16 6AE
T: 0131 666 2474
F: 0131 666 1684
E: contact@sascotland.org

**The National Association
of Farmers' Markets**
Regulates and promotes farmers'
markets. Search engine with detailed
info on local markets and good links
to other sites.
FARMA, PO Box 575
Southampton SO15 7BZ
T: 0845 230 2150
Website: www.farmersmarkets.net

BigBarn Ltd
Search for your nearest farmers'
market, farm shop, box delivery
scheme or PYO farm.
College Farm, Great Barford
Bedfordshire, MK44 3JJ
T: 01234 871005
E: ant@bigbarn.co.uk
Website: www.bigbarn.co.uk

TEAS

Try **Twinings** (www.twinings.com/)
for their green-tea blend of both black
and green teas.
Jacksons of Piccadilly (www.jacksons-of-
piccadily.com) make a calming and relaxing
organic green tea and camomile blend.
Clearspring (www.clearspring.co.uk)
produce an organic Japanese Sencha
green tea, which is used by Zen monks
to promote mental clarity and calmness
during prolonged meditations.
Clipper (www.clipper-teas.com)
manufacture an Ayurvedic Detox Infusion
which comprises an organic blend of
rosemary, ginger, oregano, turmeric,
aloe vera and lime.

BIODYNAMIC FARMS IN THE UK

Tablehurst Farm
Forest Row, East Sussex
RH18 5DP
T: 01342 823173
F: 01342 824873
E: Tablehurst_Farm@talk21.com

Hungary Lane Farm
Sutton Bonnington, Nr Loughborough
Leicestershire, LE12 5NB
T: 01509 673897

Sturts Farm and Garden
Three Cross Roads, West Moors
Ferndown, Dorset, BH22 0NF
T: 01202 870572

Garvald Home Farm
Dolphinton, West Linton, EH46 7HJ
T: 01968 682238

Plas Dwbl Farm
Plas Dwbl, Mynachlogddu
Clynderwen, Dyfed, SA66 7SE
T: 01994 419352

Pishwanton Project
Pedlar's Way, Gifford
East Lothian, EH41 4JD
T/ F: 01620 810259
E: lstrust@gn.apc.org

Botton Village Farm Training Course
Botton Village CVT, Danby
Whitby, N. Yorkshire, YO21 2NJ
T: 01287 661374
E: stormy.hall.botton@camphill.org.uk
Website:
www.camphill.org.uk/botton.htm

Ruskin Mill
Ruskin Mill College
The Fisherie, Horsley
Gloucestershire, GL6 0PL
T: 01453 837527
F: 01453 837535
E: julian.pyzer@rusk-mill.org.uk
Website: www.ruskin-mill.org.uk/

Fern Verrow
Fern Verrow, St. Margarets
Herefordshire, HR2 QF
E: fernverrow@btopenworld.com

Oaklands Park
Oaklands Park, Camphill Community
Newnham-on-Severn, Gloucestershire
GL14 1EF
T: 01594 516230
F: 01594 516821
E: cvtoaklandspark@hotmail.com
Website:
http://www.oaklandspark.org.uk

The Grange
The Grange, Camphill Community
Newnham, Gloucestershire
GL14 1HJ
T: 01594 516246
F: 01594 516 969
E: grangeoffice@phonecoop.coop

Old Plaw Hatch Farm
Sharpethorne, West Sussex,
RH19 4JL
T: 01342 810201
E: info@plawhatchfarm.co.uk

COMPLEMENTARY THERAPISTS

ACUPUNCTURE

For a list of acupuncture
practitioners, contact:

British Acupuncture Council
63 Jeddo Road, London, W12 9HQ
T: 020 8735 0400
F: 020 8735 0404
E: info@acupuncture.org.uk
Website: www.acupuncture.org.uk

ALLERGY ELIMINATION

To find an allergy therapist near
you, contact:

NAET for Europe
24 rue Carnot, 74000 Annecy, France
T: 00 33 4 50 51 31 50
F: 00 33 4 50 10 92 38
E: contact@naeteurope.com
Website: www.naeteurope.com

HYPNOTHERAPY

For a list of hypnotherapy
practitioners contact one
of the following organisations:

General Hypnotherapy Register
P O Box 204, Lymington, Hampshire
SO41 6WP
T/F: 01590 683770
E: admin@general-hypnotherapy-
register.com
Website: www.general-hypnotherapy-
register.com

The Hypnotherapy Association
14 Crown Street, Chorley
Lancashire, PR7 1DX
T: 01257 262124
F: (44) 01257 262124
E: admin@thehypnotherapy
association.co.uk
Website: www.thehypnotherapy
association.co.uk

MASSAGE AND REFLEXOLOGY

For a list of massage therapy
professional bodies and associations
visit www.massagetherapy.co.uk or email
info@massagetherapy.co.uk. To find a
qualified reflexologist in your area contact
one of the following umbrella
organisations:

Association of Reflexologists
27 Old Gloucester Street
London, WC1N 3XX
T: 0870 5673320
F: 01823 336646
E: info@aor.org.uk
Website: www.aor.org.uk

The British Reflexology Association
Administration Office, Monks Orchard
Whitbourne, Worcester, WR6 5RB
T: 01886 821207
F: 01886 822017
E: bra@britreflex.co.uk
Website: www.britreflex.co.uk

MEDITATION

For information, guidance and a list
of practitioners, contact:

British Meditation Society
PO Box 26, Chard, Somerset, TA20 2JT
T: 01460 62921

For information about transcendental
meditation visit:
www.t-m.org.uk
T: 08705 143733 between 10am and
5pm, Monday to Friday

YOGA AND PILATES

For more information about yoga and
a list of practitioners near you, contact:

British Wheel of Yoga
25 Jermyn Street, Sleaford
Lincolnshire, NG34 7RU
T: 01529 306 851
F: 01529 303 233
E: information@bwy.org.uk
Website: www.bwy.org.uk

For information about Pilates and
a list of practitioners, contact:

The Pilates Foundation UK Limited
PO Box 36052, London, SW16 1XQ
T: 07071 781 859
F: 020 8696 0088
Website: www.pilatesfoundation.com

REFERENCES

Allen, H.E., Halley-Henderson, M.A., Hass C.N. 'Chemical composition of bottled mineral water.' *Arch Environ Health*, (1989) 44, p102.

Borghi, L, et al. 'Epidemiological study of urinary tract stones in a northern Italian city.' *British Journal of Urology* (1990) 65, p231.

Evenepoel, P., Geypens, B., Luypaerts, A., Hiele, M., Ghoos, Y., & Rutgeerts, P. 'Digestibility of cooked and raw egg protein in humans as assessed by stable isotope techniques.' *Journal of Nutrition*, (1998) 128, pp1716–1722.

Hunter, P.R., Burge S.H. 'The bacteriological quality of bottled natural mineral waters.' *Epidemiol Infect* (1987) 99, p43.

Koebnick, C, Strassner C, Hoffmann I, Leitzmann C. 'Consequences of a long-term raw food diet on body weight and menstruation: results of a questionnaire survey.' *Annals of Nutrition and Metabolism*, (1999) 43, pp69–79.

Ministry of Agriculture, Fisheries and Food. *The Natural Mineral Water Regulations. Statutory Instruments No 71*. HMSO, 1985.

Rauma, A.L., Nenonen, M., Helve, T., & Hanninen, O. 'Effect of a strict vegan diet on energy and nutrient intakes by Finnish rheumatoid patients.' *European Journal of Clinical Nutrition*, (1993) 47, pp747–749.

Rauma, A.L., Torronen, R., Hanninen, O. & Mykkanen, H. 'Vitamin B-12 status of long-term adherents of a strict uncooked vegan diet ("living food diet") is compromised.' *Journal of Nutrition*, (1995) 125, pp2511–2515.

Walker, A. 'Drinking water – doubts about quality.' *Br Med J*, (1992) 304, p 175.

INDEX

Figures in bold indicate main references.